ENT

AN INTRODUCTION
AND PRACTICAL GUIDE

SECOND EDITION

ENT

AN INTRODUCTION
AND PRACTICAL GUIDE

SECOND EDITION

EDITED BY

James Russell Tysome MA PhD FRCS (ORL-HNS)
Consultant ENT and Skull Base Surgeon
Cambridge University Hospitals NHS Foundation Trust

AND

Rahul Govind Kanegaonkar FRCS (ORL-HNS)
Consultant ENT Surgeon
Medway NHS Foundation Trust

Visiting Professor in Otorhinolaryngology
Professor of Medical Innovation
Canterbury Christ Church University

CRC Press
Taylor & Francis Group
Boca Raton London New York

CRC Press is an imprint of the
Taylor & Francis Group, an **informa** business

CRC Press
Taylor & Francis Group
6000 Broken Sound Parkway NW, Suite 300
Boca Raton, FL 33487-2742

International Standard Book Number-13: 978-1-138-19823-4 (Paperback)

Library of Congress Cataloging-in-Publication Data

Names: Tysome, James Russell, author. | Kanegaonkar, Rahul Govind, author.
Title: ENT : an introduction and practical guide / [edited by] James Tysome, Rahul Kanegaonkar.
Description: Second edition. | Boca Raton, FL : CRC Press, Taylor & Francis Group, 2018. | Includes bibliographical references and index.
Identifiers: LCCN 2017019190 (print) | LCCN 2017019740 (ebook) |
ISBN 9781315270524 (General eBook) | ISBN 9781351982337 (Adobe eBook) |
ISBN 9781351982320 (ePub eBook) | ISBN 9781351982313 (Mobipocket eBook) |
ISBN 9781138298149 (hardback : alk. paper) | ISBN 9781138198234 (pbk. : alk. paper)
Subjects: | MESH: Otorhinolaryngologic Surgical Procedures--methods |
Otorhinolaryngologic Diseases--surgery
Classification: LCC RF46.5 (ebook) | LCC RF46.5 (print) | NLM WV 168 | DDC 617.5/1--dc23
LC record available at https://lccn.loc.gov/2017019190

Visit the Taylor & Francis Web site at
http://www.taylorandfrancis.com

and the CRC Press Web site at
http://www.crcpress.com

Printed and bound in the United States of America by
Edwards Brothers Malloy on sustainably sourced paper

Dedication
This book is dedicated to Dipalee, Amee and Deven,
and to Laura, George, Henry and Max

CONTENTS

FOREWORD

The 'Introduction to ENT' course has now become an established and must-attend course for the novice ENT practitioner. The synergistic blend of didactic teaching and practical skills training has allowed many junior trainees to raise the standard of care that they deliver to their ENT patients.

The course manual is now a 'Bible' for junior students in nursing and medicine, caring for patients on wards, clinics or in emergency rooms. The Royal College of Surgeons has endorsed this course in the past and it continues to maintain a high standard for postgraduate training. I strongly recommend this course to any trainee embarking on a career in ENT.

Khalid Ghufoor
Otolaryngology Tutor
Raven Department of Education
The Royal College of Surgeons of England

PREFACE

This book has been written for trainees in otorhinolaryngology and to update general practitioners. Common and significant pathology that might present itself is described. Included also are relevant supporting specialties such as audiology and radiology. A significant proportion of this text has been devoted to common surgical procedures, their indications and operative techniques, as well as to the management of their complications. We do hope that the text will facilitate and encourage junior trainees to embark on a career in this diverse and rewarding specialty.

Writing this book would not have been possible had it not been for the encouragement of our many friends and colleagues, and the unfaltering support of our families.

We would, however, like to make a special mention of some extraordinary and gifted tutors without whom we might neither have initiated the popular 'Introduction to ENT' course nor written the course manual from which this text originates. Ghassan Alusi, Alec Fitzgerald O'Connor, Khalid Ghufoor, Govind Kanegaonkar, Robert Tranter and the late Roger Parker instilled in us a passion for teaching, nurtured our curiosity for all things medical and encouraged us to undertake the research that has served us so well.

James R Tysome and Rahul G Kanegaonkar

INTRODUCTION

Otorhinolaryngology (ENT) is a diverse and challenging specialty. It is often poorly represented in busy medical school curriculums and specialty optionals at some Universities. Although an estimated 20% of cases seen in primary care are ENT related, many general practitioners have little or no formal training in this specialty.

This second edition has been revised and updated to reflect recent advances in Otorhinolaryngology.

This book has evolved from the 'Introduction to ENT' course manual, which has served many of us so well. Over 3000 doctors have attended this course and its 'Essential Guide' counterpart.

This book covers both common and uncommon, including life-threatening emergencies that may present themselves in both primary and secondary care. Management pathways are described as are commonly performed surgical procedures and possible complications. This book further provides a basis for referral if required.

The updated colour illustrations concisely depict relevant clinical anatomy without unduly simplifying the topic in question.

I am certain that this current text will prove to be as, if not more, popular and relevant to general practitioners than the 'Introduction to ENT' text from which it is derived.

Dr Junaid Bajwa
October 2016

CONTRIBUTORS

Mr Ketan Desai FRCS
Associate Specialist in Otorhinolaryngologist
Royal Sussex County Hospital, Brighton, UK

Mr Neil Donnelly MSc (HONS) FRCS (ORL-HNS)
Consultant Otoneurological and Skull Base Surgeon
Cambridge University Hospitals NHS Foundation Trust, Cambridge, UK

Dr Dipalee Durve MRCPCH and FRCR
Consultant Radiologist
Guy's and St Thomas' NHS Foundation Trust, London, UK

Mr James Tysome MA PhD FRCS (ORL-HNS)
Consultant ENT and Skull Base Surgeon
Cambridge University Hospitals NHS Foundation Trust, Cambridge, UK

Professor Rahul Kanegaonkar FRCS (ORL-HNS)
Consultant ENT Surgeon
Medway NHS Foundation Trust, Gillingham, UK

and

Visiting Professor in Otorhinolaryngology
Professor of Medical Innovation
Canterbury Christ Church University, Canterbury, UK

Dr Olivia Kenyon
ENT Senior House Officer
Cambridge University Hospitals, Cambridge, UK

Ms Sonia Kumar FRCS (ORL-HNS)
Fellow in Paediatric Otolaryngology
Great Ormond Street Hospital for Sick Children, London, UK

Dr Kaggere Paramesh
Specialist Registrar in Radiology
Guy's and St Thomas' NHS Foundation Trust, London, UK

Mr Ram Moorthy FRCS (ORL-HNS)
Consultant ENT Surgeon
Heatherwood and Wexham Park Hospitals NHS Foundation Trust and
Honorary Consultant ENT Surgeon, Northwick Park Hospital, London, UK

Ms Joanne Rimmer FRCS (ORL-HNS)
Consultant ENT Surgeon/Rhinologist, Monash Health
Honorary Senior Lecturer, Monash University, Melbourne, Australia

Professor Francis Vaz FRCS (ORL-HNS)
Consultant ENT/Head and Neck Surgeon
University College London Hospital, London, UK

Mr Max Whittaker FRCS (ORL-HNS)
Specialist Registrar in Otorhinolaryngology
Kent, Surrey and Sussex Deanery, London, UK

1 CLINICAL ANATOMY

Max Whittaker

THE EAR

The ear is a highly specialized organ dedicated to the detection of both sound and head movement. It is classically described as three separate but functionally related subunits. The outer ear, consisting of the pinna and external auditory canal, is bounded medially by the lateral surface of the tympanic membrane. The middle ear contains the ossicular chain, which spans the middle ear cleft and enables the transfer of acoustic energy from the tympanic membrane to the oval window. The inner ear comprises both the cochlea, which converts mechanical vibrations to electrical impulses in the auditory nerve, and the vestibular apparatus.

The pinna acts to direct sound into the external auditory canal, and plays an important role in sound localization. It consists predominantly of an elastic cartilaginous framework over which the skin is tightly adherent (Figure 1.1). The cartilage is dependent on a sheet of overlying perichondrium for its nutritional support; hence separation of this layer by a haematoma, abscess or inflammation secondary to piercing may result in cartilage necrosis and permanent deformity (cauliflower ear). The lobule, in contrast, is a well-vascularized fibrofatty skin tag.

The pinna develops from six mesodermal condensations, the hillocks of His, as early as the sixth embryological week. Three hillocks arise

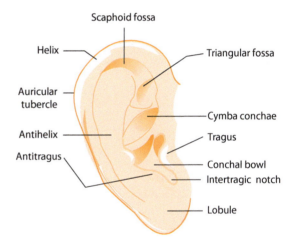

Figure 1.1. Surface landmarks of the pinna.

from each of the first and second branchial arches on either side of the first pharyngeal groove. These rotate and fuse to produce an elaborate but surprisingly consistent structure. Incomplete fusion may result in an accessory auricle or pre-auricular sinus, while failure of development of the antihelix (from the fourth hillock) in a protruding or 'bat' ear.

The external auditory canal is a tortuous passage that redirects and redistributes sound from the conchal bowl to the tympanic membrane. The skin of the lateral third of the external auditory canal is thick, contains ceruminous glands, is hair-bearing and tightly adherent to the underlying fibrocartilage.

In contrast, the skin of the medial two-thirds is thin, hairless, tightly bound to underlying bone and exquisitely sensitive.

The sensory nerve supply of the canal is largely provided by the auriculotemporal and greater auricular nerves. There are minor contributions from the facial nerve (hence vesicles arise on the posterolateral surface of the canal as seen in Ramsay Hunt syndrome) and Arnold's nerve, a branch of the vagus nerve (provoking the cough reflex when stimulated with a cotton bud or during microsuction). The squamous epithelium of the tympanic membrane and ear canal is unique and deserves a special mention. The superficial layer of keratin of the skin of the ear is shed laterally during maturation. This produces an escalator

mechanism that allows debris to be directed out of the canal. Disruption of this mechanism may result in debris accumulation, recurrent infections (otitis externa) or erosion of the ear canal, as seen in keratitis obturans.

The tympanic membrane is bounded circumferentially by the annulus, and is continuous with the posterior wall of the ear canal. It consists of three layers: laterally, a squamous epithelial layer; a middle layer of collagen fibres providing tensile strength; and a medial surface lined with respiratory epithelium continuous with the middle ear.

The 80 mm^2 of the tympanic membrane surface area is divided into pars tensa, accounting for the majority, approximately 55 mm^2, and pars flaccida, or attic (Figure 1.2). These regions are structurally and functionally different. The collagen fibres of

Figure 1.2. Right tympanic membrane.

Labels (left): Chorda tympani; Long process of incus; Umbo; Round window niche

Labels (right): Scutum; Pars flaccida; Lateral process of malleus; Handle of malleus; Pars tensa; Eustachian tube; Light reflex; Promontory

the pars tensa are arranged as lateral radial fibres and medial circumferential fibres that distort the membrane. As a result, the pars tensa 'billows' laterally from the malleus and buckles when presented with sound, conducting acoustic energy to the ossicular chain. In contrast, the collagen fibres of the pars flaccida are randomly scattered and this section is relatively flat. Interestingly, high-frequency sounds preferentially alter the

posterior half of the tympanic membrane, while low-frequency sounds alter the anterior half.

The handle and lateral process of the malleus are embedded within the tympanic membrane and firmly adherent at the umbo ("Lloyd's ligament"). The long process of the incus is also commonly seen, although the heads of the ossicles are hidden behind the thin bone of the scutum superiorly.

The middle ear

The middle ear is an irregular, air-filled space containing the three ossicles: the malleus, incus and stapes. Its predominant function is to overcome impedance mismatch, energy lost when transferring sound from one medium to another, in this case converting air vibrations at the tympanic membrane to fluid vibrations within the cochlea. The ossicular chain is crucial in this process, by conducting vibrations to the cochlea via the stapes footplate at the oval window. Without it the vast majority of acoustic energy would not be transmitted through the oval window resulting in a conductive hearing loss of up to 50–60 dB. Clinically, ossicular discontinuity or fixation of the footplate by otosclerosis prevents sound conduction to the inner ear, resulting in a conductive hearing loss.

The middle ear mechanisms that improve sound transfer include:

- The relative ratios of the areas of the tympanic membrane to stapes footplate (17:1).
- The relative lengths of the handle of malleus to the long process of incus (1.3:1).
- The natural resonance of the outer and middle ears.
- The phase difference between the oval and round windows.
- The buckling effect of the tympanic membrane (2:1).

In combination the total margin of improvement amounts to 44:1.

In order to optimise admittance, middle ear air pressure is equalized with atmospheric pressure. This is achieved via the Eustachian tube, which communicates with the nasopharynx, and opens on chewing, swallowing and yawning, allowing air to pass into the middle ear cleft (Figure 1.3). The amount of air passing through the Eustachian tube varies greatly between individuals depending on pressure gradient and volume of the mastoid air cell system; however, it is thought that the equalisation process occurs rapidly, between 0.15 and 0.34 seconds. In children, Eustachian tube dysfunction is common and may result in negative

Aditus (inlet) to mastoid antrum

Malleus

Incus

Chordo tympani

Tensor of tympani

Tendon of stapedius

Tympanic membrane

Facial n. (CN VII) in facial canal

Prominence of lateral semicircular canal

Prominence of facial canal

Stapes

Promontory

Tympanic plexus

Tympanic n.

Figure 1.3. Coronal section of the ossicles in the middle ear.

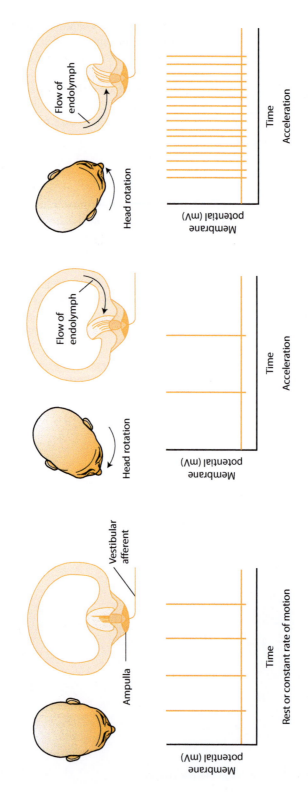

Figure 1.4. The inner ear. Angular acceleration is detected by the ampullae of the lateral semicircular canals, while linear acceleration and static head tilt are detected by the maculae of the utricle and saccule.

middle ear pressure, recurrent otitis media or middle ear effusions.

■ The inner ear

The inner ear consists of the cochlea and peripheral vestibular apparatus (Figure 1.4).

The cochlea is a two and three-quarter-turn snail shell that houses the organ of Corti. It is tonotopically arranged, with high frequencies detected at the base and low frequencies nearest the apical turn. Acoustic energy presented at the oval window causes a travelling wave along the basilar membrane, with maximal deflection at a frequency-specific region of the cochlea. This results in depolarization of the inner hair cells at this region, and through a process of mechanotransduction, vibrational energy is converted to neural impulses relayed centrally via the cochlear nerve.

The peripheral vestibular system is responsible for the detection of head movement. While the semicircular canals are stimulated by rotational acceleration, the saccule and utricle are dedicated to detecting static and linear head movements. This is achieved by two similar, but functionally different sensory receptor systems (Figure 1.4).

The semicircular canals are oriented in orthogonal planes to one another and organized into functional pairs: the two horizontal semicircular canals working in tandem, and the superior canals paired with the contralateral posterior canals.

The sensory neuroepithelium of the semicircular canals is limited to a dilated segment of the bony and membranous labyrinth, the ampulla. Within this region, a crest perpendicular to the long axis of each canal bears a mound of connective tissue from which projects a layer of hair cells. Their cilia insert into a gelatinous mass, the cupula, which is deflected during rotational head movements.

Within the utricle and saccule, the sensory patches, called maculae are orientated in order to detect linear acceleration and head tilt in horizontal and vertical planes, respectively. Hair cells in these maculae are arranged in an elaborate manner and project into a fibro-calcareous sheet, the otoconial membrane. As this membrane has a greater specific gravity than the surrounding endolymph, head tilt and linear movement result in the otoconial membrane moving relative to the underlying hair cells. The shearing force produced causes depolarization of the underlying hair cells with conduction centrally through the inferior and superior vestibular nerves.

THE FACIAL NERVE

The facial nerve (CN VII) runs a tortuous course from the brainstem, through the temporal bone before exiting the skull base at the stylomastoid foramen and dividing within the parotid gland (Figure 1.5). Therefore, disease processes affecting the inner ear, middle ear, skull base or parotid gland may result in facial nerve paralysis.

The facial nerve arises from three nuclei in the brainstem: the motor nucleus, superior salivatory nucleus in the pons, and the nucleus solitarius in the medulla. During its intracranial segment branches from the latter two nuclei join to form the nervus intermedius carrying parasympathetic and sensory fibres. These are joined at the internal acoustic canal by the motor fibres to form the facial nerve, running anterosuperiorly through the meatal segment in relation to the vestibulocochlear nerve. In the labyrinthine segment the nerve undergoes a posterior deflection at the first genu, in close relation to the geniculate ganglion, housing the cell bodies of the chorda tympani, and the greater superficial petrosal nerve exits via the facial hiatus to supply the lacrimal gland. The facial nerve passes along its tympanic horizontal portion within the medial

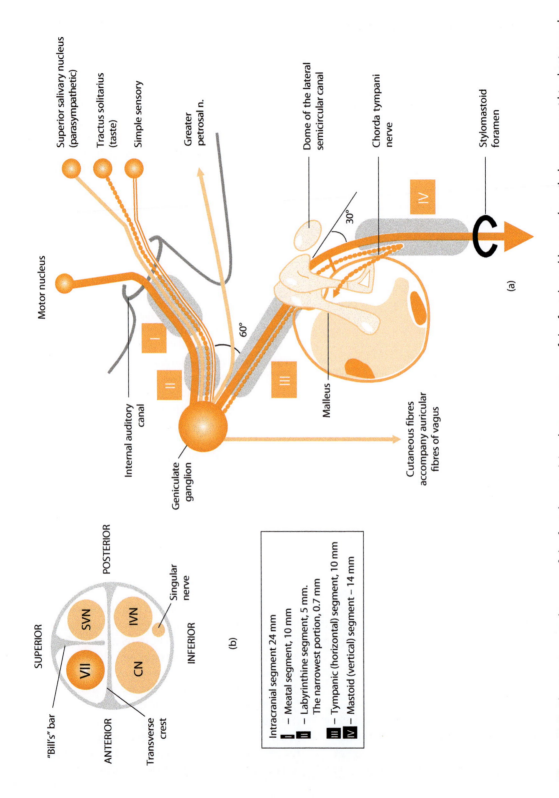

Figure 1.5. The intratemporal course of the facial nerve (a), relative positions of the facial, cochlear and vestibular nerves within the internal auditory canal (b). (VII = facial nerve, SVN = superior vestibular nerve, IVN = inferior vestibular nerve.)

Superior salivary nucleus (parasympathetic)

Tractus solitarius (taste)

Simple sensory

Greater petrosal n.

Dome of the lateral semicircular canal

Chorda tympani nerve

Stylomastoid foramen

Motor nucleus

Internal auditory canal

Geniculate ganglion

Malleus

Cutaneous fibres accompany auricular fibres of vagus

60°

30°

I

II

III

IV

C

(a)

SUPERIOR

POSTERIOR

"Bill's" bar

SVN

IVN

Singular nerve

VII

CN

ANTERIOR

INFERIOR

Transverse crest

(b)

Intracranial segment 24 mm
 – Meatal segment, 10 mm
 – Labyrinthine segment, 5 mm.
   The narrowest portion, 0.7 mm
 – Tympanic (horizontal) segment, 10 mm
 – Mastoid (vertical) segment – 14 mm

III

IV

wall of the middle ear to the second genu. At this point it undergoes a further deflection inferiorly to begin its vertical mastoid segment. Motor branches are given off to stapedius and taste fibres from the anterior two-thirds of the tongue are received from the chorda tympani.

The facial nerve exits the skull base at the stylomastoid foramen to begin its extratemporal course, and adopts a more variable anatomy. Lying in the tympanomastoid groove it courses anteriorly to enter the parotid gland, where it most commonly forms superior and inferior divisions before terminating in its five motor branches (Figure 1.6). Additional branches supply the posterior belly of digastric and stylohyoid muscles.

Figure 1.6. External branches of the facial nerve.

THE NOSE

The nose and nasal cavity serve a number of functions. While their principal function is provision of an airway, secondary functions include:

- Warming of inspired air.
- Humidification of inspired air.
- Filtering of large particulate matter by coarse hairs (the vibrissiae) in the nasal vestibule.
- Mucus production, trapping and ciliary clearance of particulate matter.
- Immune protection (within mucus and via presentation to the adenoidal pad).

- Olfaction.
- Drainage and aeration of the middle ear cleft via the Eustachian tube.
- Drainage and aeration of the paranasal sinuses.
- Drainage for the nasolacrimal duct.
- Prevention of lung alveolar collapse via the nasal cycle.
- Voice modification.
- Pheromone detection via the Vomeronasal organ of Jacobsen.

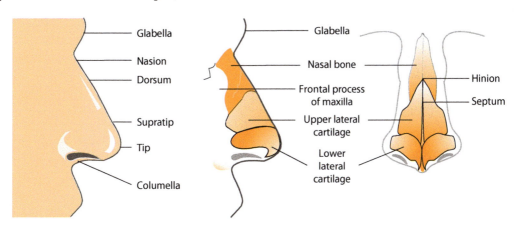

Figure 1.7. Nasal landmarks and external nasal skeleton.

▌ Nasal skeleton

The external nasal skeleton consists of bone in the upper third (the nasal bones) and cartilage in the lower two-thirds. External nasal landmarks are illustrated in Figure 1.7 and ensure accurate description when assessing the nose prior to considering surgical intervention.

▌ The nasal cavities

The nasal cavities are partitioned in the midline by the nasal septum, which consists of both fibrocartilage and bone (Figure 1.8).

As with the cartilage of the pinna, the cartilage of the septum is dependent on the overlying

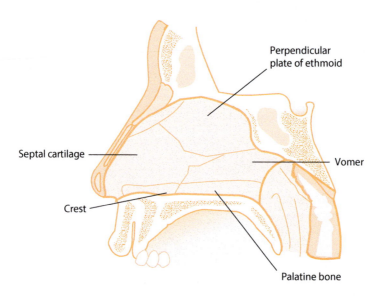

Figure 1.8. The skeleton of the nasal septum.

adherent perichondrium for its nutritional support. Separation of this layer by haematoma or abscess may result in cartilage necrosis, perforation and a saddle nose deformity.

In contrast to the smooth surface of the nasal septum, the surface of the lateral wall is thrown into folds by three bony projections: the inferior, middle and superior turbinates (Figure 1.9). These highly vascular structures become cyclically engorged resulting in alternating increased airway resistance and reduced airflow from one nasal cavity to the other over a period of 2–3 hours. This physiological process, under hypothalamic control, may be more noticeable in patients with a septal deviation or in those with rhinitis.

The nasal cavity has a rich blood supply originating from both the internal and external carotid arteries (Figure 1.10). As a result, epistaxis may result in considerable blood loss which should not be underestimated. In cases of intractable posterior nasal bleeding, the sphenopalatine artery may be endoscopically ligated by raising a mucoperiosteal flap on the lateral nasal wall. Bleeding from the ethmoidal vessels requires a periorbital incision and identification of these vessels as they pass from the orbital cavity into the nasal cavity in the fronto-ethmoidal suture.

The venous drainage of the nose and mid-face communicates with the cavernous sinus of the middle cranial fossa via the superior ophthalmic

Figure 1.9. The lateral surface of the nasal cavity.

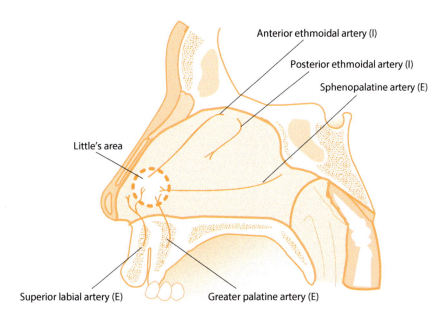

Figure 1.10. Arterial blood supply to the nose. The nose has a rich blood supply, supplied by both internal (I) and external (E) carotid arteries.

vein, or deep facial vein and pterygoid plexus. As a result, infection in this territory may spread intracranially, resulting in cavernous sinus thrombosis and may be life-threatening.

The olfactory mucosa is limited to a superior region of the nasal cavity (Figure 1.9). Once dissolved in mucus, olfactants combine with binding proteins and stimulate specific olfactory bipolar cells.

Their axons converge to produce 12–20 olfactory bundles, which relay information centrally to secondary neurones within the olfactory bulbs at the cribriform fossae of the anterior cranial fossa.

The paranasal sinuses are paired air-filled spaces that communicate with the nasal cavity via ostia located on the lateral nasal wall (Figure 1.11). These occur at different ages, with the maxillary sinuses

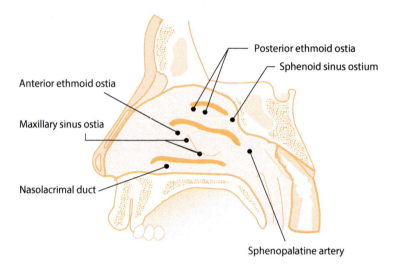

Figure 1.11. The lateral wall of the nasal cavity. (The turbinates have been removed in order to allow visualization of the ostia of the paranasal sinuses.)

present at birth and the frontal sinuses being the last to fully form. In a minority of patients the frontal sinuses may be entirely absent. Mucus produced by the respiratory epithelium within the paranasal sinuses does not drain entirely by gravity. In the maxillary sinus, for example, cilliary activity

results in a spiral flow that directs mucus up and medially to the ostium high on the medial wall.

The anterior and posterior ethmoidal air cells are separated from the orbital contents by the lamina papyracea, a thin plate of bone derived from the

Figure 1.12. Coronal section of the paranasal sinuses.

ethmoid bone. Infection within these paranasal sinuses may extend laterally through this layer, resulting in periorbital cellulitis and possible loss of vision.

The osteomeatal complex represents a region through which the paranasal sinuses drain (Figure 1.12). Obstruction may lead to acute or chronic sinusitis; hence opening this area is pivotal when surgically treating sinus disease.

ORAL CAVITY

The oral cavity is bounded anteriorly by the lips, posteriorly by the anterior tonsillar pillars, inferiorly by the tongue base and superiorly by the hard and soft palates (Figure 1.13).

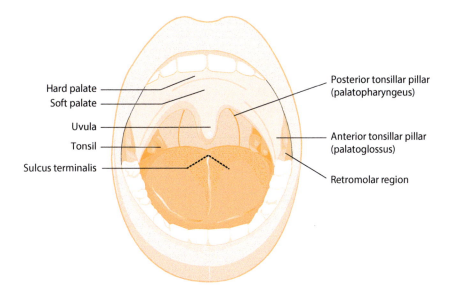

Figure 1.13. The oral cavity.

The tongue consists of a mass of striated muscle separated in the midline by a fibrous membrane. Both the intrinsic muscles (contained entirely within the tongue) and the extrinsic muscles (inserted into bone) are supplied by the hypoglossal nerve, except for the palatoglossus (supplied by the pharyngeal plexus). A unilateral hypoglossal nerve palsy results in deviation of the tongue towards the side of the weakness.

The tongue is derived from the mesoderm of the first four branchial arches. Its embryological origin is reflected in its pattern of innervation, and arrangement of the fungiform, foliate, circumvallate and filiform papillae on its dorsal surface. The anterior two thirds, formed from the first arch, are coated by fungiform papillae, which distinguish the five tastes: sweet, salty, sour, bitter and umami. These are interspersed with the filiform papillae which do not contribute to taste but act to increase surface area, providing friction and enabling manipulation of food. Taste receptors are innervated by the chorda tympani, which hitchhikes with the lingual nerve to join the facial nerve. The mandibular branch of the trigeminal nerve supplies touch and temperature sensation.

The posterior third is predominantly derived from the third and fourth arches, with a small contribution from the second. Its surface is lined laterally by foliate papillae, with taste, touch and temperature sensation relayed by the glossopharyngeal and superior laryngeal nerves.

These two distinct regions are separated by a row of circumvallate papillae in the form of an inverted 'V'. The foramen caecum lies at the apex of this 'V' and represents the site of embryological origin of the thyroid gland (see below). Rarely, due to failure of migration, a lingual thyroid may present as a mass at this site.

The floor of the mouth is separated from the neck by the mylohyoid muscle. The muscle fans out from the lateral border of the hyoid bone to insert into the medial surface of the mandible as far back as the second molar tooth. A dental root infection that is anterior to this may result in an abscess forming in the floor of the mouth (Ludwig's angina). This is a potentially life-threatening airway emergency and requires urgent intervention to extract the affected tooth and drain the abscess.

The hyoid bone lies at the level of the third cervical vertebra. The larynx is suspended from this C-shaped bone, resulting in the rise of the laryngeal skeleton during swallowing.

THE PHARYNX

The pharynx consists of a curved fibrous sheet, the pharyngobasilar fascia, enclosed within three stacked muscular bands: the superior, middle and inferior constrictors. The muscle fibres of the constrictors sweep posteriorly and medially to meet in a midline posterior raphe. The pharyngeal plexus provides the motor supply to the musculature of the pharynx, except for the stylopharyngeus which is supplied by the glossopharyngeal nerve.

The superior constrictor arises from the medial pterygoid plate, hamulus, pterygomandibluar raphe and mandible. The Eustachian tube passes between its superior border and the skull base. Stylopharyngeus and the glossopharyngeal and lingual nerves pass below the constrictor.

The middle constrictor arises from the greater horn of the hyoid bone, its fibres sweeping to enclose the superior constrictor (as low as the vocal cords).

The inferior constrictor consists of two striated muscles, the thyropharyngeus and cricopharyngeus. A potential area of weakness lies between the two muscles posteriorly: Killian's dehiscence. A pulsion divertivulum may form a pharyngeal pouch at this site, leading to retention and regurgitation of ingested material.

The upper aero-digestive tract is divided into the nasal cavity and nasopharynx, oral cavity and oropharynx, larynx and hypopharynx (Figure 1.14).

The nasopharynx extends from the skull base to the soft palate. It communicates with the middle ear cleft via the Eustachian tube (Figure 1.15). This tube unwinds during yawning and chewing, allowing air to pass into the middle ear cleft and maintaining atmospheric pressure within the middle ear. This mechanism depends on the actions of levator and tensor veli palatini muscles, hence a cleft palate is often associated with chronic Eustachian tube dysfunction. Equally, blockage of the Eustachian tube may result in a middle ear effusion. Whilst effusions are common in children, unilateral effusions in adults should raise suspicion of post-nasal space pathology, such as a nasopharyngeal carcinoma arising from the fossa of Rossenmüller. The adenoid gland lies on the posterior nasopharyngeal wall, forming part of Waldeyers ring of immune tissue, along with the palatine and lingual tonsils. Adenoid enlargement may compromise airflow resulting in obstructive sleep apnoea, and may require surgical reduction.

The oropharynx spans from the soft palate to the level of the epiglottis. Its lateral walls are formed by the palatoglossus and palatopharyngeus muscles, between which lie the palatine tonsils. These receive a rich blood supply from the lingual, facial and ascending pharyngeal branches of the external carotid artery.

Figure 1.14. Sagittal section through the head and neck. Note the hard palate lies at C1, the hyoid bone at C3 and the cricoid cartilage at C6.

Figure 1.15. Endoscopic view of the right postnasal space.

The laryngopharynx lies posterior to the larynx. It is bounded inferiorly by the cricoids, where the cricopharyngeus marks the transition into the oesophagus.

THE LARYNX

The principal function of the larynx is that of a protective sphincter preventing aspiration of ingested material (Figure 1.16). Phonation is a secondary function. The three single cartilages of the larynx are the epiglottic, thyroid and cricoid cartilages. The three paired cartilages of the larynx

- Interarytenoid bar
- Right arytenoid
- Cricoid cartilage
- Right vocal cord
- Quadrangular membrane
- Epiglottis
- Median glossoepiglottic fold
- Posterior pharyngeal wall
- Left pyriform fossa
- Laryngeal inlet
- Left vallecula
- Lingual tonsil

Figure 1.16. Endoscopic view of the larynx.

are the arytenoid, corniculate and cuneiform cartilages.

The arytenoid cartilages are pyramidal structures from which the vocal cords project forward and medially. Abduction (lateral movement) of the cords is dependent on the posterior cricoarytenoid muscle, hence this is described as the most important muscle of the larynx. Additional instrinsic and extrinsic muscles provide adduction and variable cord tension.

The motor supply of the muscles of the larynx is derived from the recurrent laryngeal nerves. An ipsilateral palsy results in hoarseness, while a bilateral palsy results in stridor and airway obstruction.

The cricoid is a signet ring-shaped structure which supports the arytenoid cartilages. As the only complete ring of cartilage in the airway, trauma may cause oedema and obstruction of the central lumen.

The formula describes airflow through the lumen of a tube (Figure 1.17).

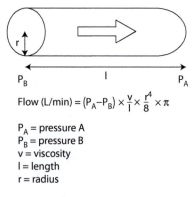

$$\text{Flow (L/min)} = (P_A - P_B) \times \frac{v}{l} \times \frac{r^4}{8} \times \pi$$

P_A = pressure A
P_B = pressure B
v = viscosity
l = length
r = radius

Figure 1.17. Flow through a tube.

Reducing the lumen of a tube by half causes the flow to fall to 1/16 of the original. Therefore, relatively minor oedema may result in a dramatic reduction in airflow.

THE THYROID AND PARATHYROID GLANDS

The thyroid is an endocrine gland, producing thyroid hormone under hypothalamic–pituitary control. It consists of two lobes connected by an isthmus, and a variably-sized pyramidal lobe. Its blood supply is derived from superior and inferior thyroid arteries, and occasionally the thyroid ima artery running directly from the brachiocephalic trunk or right common carotid artery. Venous drainage is achieved via the superior, middle and inferior thyroid veins.

The gland develops embryologically at the tongue base during weeks 3–4 and progresses inferiorly anterior to the pharynx along the thyroglossal duct to occupy its final position over the 2nd and 3rd tracheal rings. Failure of degeneration of this duct may result in formation of a thyroglossal cyst presenting as a midline neck mass, which, due to its origins, clinically rises on tongue protrusion.

The four parathyroid glands also perform an endocrine function, producing parathyroid hormone and calcitonin involved in calcium regulation. The two inferior glands originate from the 3rd branchial pouch and migrate inferiorly to occupy variable positions in the neck. As such, their blood supply is equally variable, but most frequently via the inferior thyroid arteries. The superior glands are formed by the 4th branchial pouch. Lying in close proximity to the thyroid, their blood supply is derived from the inferior thyroid arteries.

THE MAJOR SALIVARY GLANDS

Whilst minor salivary glands are scattered within the oral cavity, saliva is predominantly produced by three paired major salivary glands: the parotid, submandibular and sublingual glands (Figure 1.18).

The parotid gland is a large, serous salivary gland enclosed by an extension of the investing layer of deep fascia of the neck. This parotid fascia is unforgiving, and inflammation of the gland may result in severe pain.

Saliva produced by the parotid gland drains via Stensen's duct. The duct is approximately 5 cm in length and lies superficial to the masseter muscle. At the anterior border of this muscle it pierces the fibres of the buccinator to enter the oral cavity opposite the upper 2nd molar tooth.

The facial nerve passes into and divides within the substance of the parotid gland to separate it into superficial and deep portions. Hence, an abscess or malignant lesion within the parotid gland may result in facial paralysis.

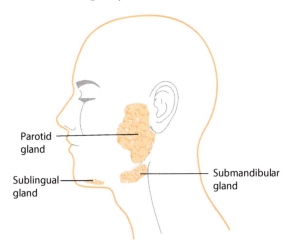

Figure 1.18. The major salivary glands of the head and neck.

In addition, the retromandibular vein passes through the anterior portion of the gland and is a useful radiological marker for defining the superficial and deep portions of the gland.

The submandibular gland is a mixed serous and mucous salivary gland and forms the majority of saliva production at rest. Its superficial portion fills the space between the mandible and mylohyoid muscle, while its deep part lies between the mylohyoid and hyoglossus. The gland drains into the floor of the oral cavity via Wharton's duct, the papilla lying adjacent to the lingual frenulum. The duct may become obstructed by a calculus, which causes painful enlargement of the gland.

The sublingual glands lie anterior to hyoglossus in the sublingual fossa of the mandible. These mucus glands drain via multiple openings into the submandibular duct and sublingual fold of the floor of the oral cavity.

CERVICAL LYMPH NODES

The neck is divided into levels 1–6, which describe groups of lymph nodes. The landmarks are:

Level 1 – Submental and submandibular triangles, bounded by the midline, digastric and the mandible.
Level 2 – Anterior triangle including sternocleidomastoid from skull base to the inferior border of hyoid.
Level 3 – Anterior triangle including sternocleidomastoid from inferior border of hyoid to inferior border of cricoid.
Level 4 – Anterior triangle including sternocleidomastoid from inferior border of cricoid to superior border of clavicle.
Level 5 – Posterior triangle: lateral border of sternocleidomastoid, superior border of clavicle, medial border of trapezius.
Level 6 – Paratracheal lymph nodes medial to the carotid.

These levels allow description of the various types of neck dissection that are performed when managing malignant disease (Figure 1.19). For example, a modified radical neck dissection involves removal of levels 1–5.

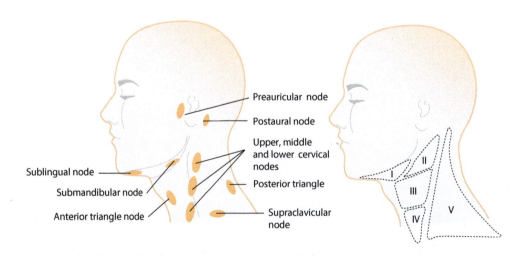

Figure 1.19. Lymph nodes groups and the triangles of the neck.

SENSORY DISTRIBUTION OF THE FACE

The sensory nerve supply of the face is derived from branches of the trigeminal nerve (Figure 1.20). Herpes zoster reactivation will result in a pattern of vesicular eruption consistent with the distribution of that division.

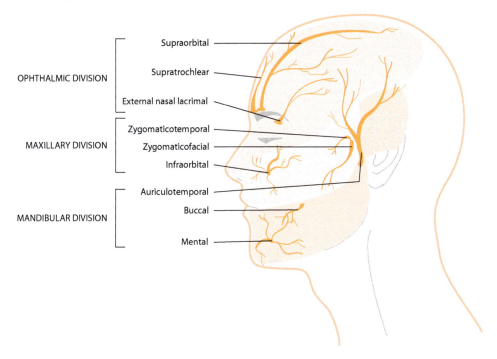

OPHTHALMIC DIVISION
- Supraorbital
- Supratrochlear
- External nasal lacrimal

MAXILLARY DIVISION
- Zygomaticotemporal
- Zygomaticofacial
- Infraorbital

MANDIBULAR DIVISION
- Auriculotemporal
- Buccal
- Mental

Figure 1.20. Sensory distribution of the face.

DEEP NECK SPACES

A thorough anatomical understanding of the deep neck spaces is crucial in identifying and managing complications of oropharyngeal infections.

The parapharyngeal space is a potential space in the form of an inverted pyramid running from the skull base to the greater cornu of the hyoid, bounded by the pharynx medially, pterygomandibular raphe anteriorly and mandible laterally. It is divided into two compartments:

- *Prestyloid* – Containing maxillary artery, inferior alveolar, lingual and auriculotemporal nerves and fat.

- *Poststyloid* – Containing carotid artery, internal jugular vein, sympathetic chain and cranial nerves IX, X and XI.

Peritonsillar or dental infections may spread along this space to form parapharyngeal abscesses requiring urgent drainage.

The retropharyngeal space is a midline potential space between the alar and prevertebral faciae, extending from the skull base to the mediastinum. It contains lymphatics draining the nasal and oral cavities, oropharynx and nasopharynx. As such it represents a path of least resistance for infection to spread to the intrathoracic compartment leading to mediastinitis.

2

ENT EXAMINATION

Ketan Desai

A thorough clinical examination is essential in the diagnosis and management of every patient.

This chapter provides a systematic and thorough stepwise guide for clinicians assessing patients.

OTOSCOPY

Ensure that both you and the patient are seated comfortably and at the same level.

Examine the pinna, postaural region and adjacent scalp for scars, discharge, swelling and any skin lesions or defects (Figure 2.1). Choose the largest speculum that will fit comfortably into the ear and place it onto the otoscope.

Gently pull the pinna upwards and backwards to straighten the ear canal (backwards in children). Infection or inflammation may cause this manoeuvre to be painful.

Hold the otoscope like a pen and rest your small digit on the patient's zygomatic arch. Any unexpected head movement will now push the

Site of endaural incision

Site of postaural incision

Figure 2.1. Examination of the pinna and postaural region. The pinna is pulled up and back and the tragus pushed forward in order to straighten the external auditory canal during otoscopy.

speculum away from the ear, preventing trauma. Use the light to observe the direction of the ear canal and the tympanic membrane. The eardrum is better visualized by using the left hand for the left ear and the right hand for the right ear. Insert the speculum gently into the meatus, pushing the tragus forward. This further straightens the ear canal.

Inspect the entrance of the canal as you insert the speculum. Pass the tip through the hairs of the canal but no further. Looking through the otoscope, examine the ear canal and tympanic membrane (Figure 2.2). Adjust your position and the otoscope to view all of the tympanic membrane in a systematic manner. The ear cannot be judged to be normal until all areas of the tympanic membrane are viewed: the handle of malleus, pars tensa, pars flaccida (or attic) and anterior recess. If the view of the tympanic membrane is obscured by the presence of wax, this must be removed. If the patient has undergone mastoid surgery where the posterior ear canal wall has been removed, methodically inspect all parts of the cavity and tympanic membrane or drum remnant by adjusting your position. The normal appearance of a mastoid cavity varies; practice and experience will allow you to recognize pathology.

Figure 2.2. Examination of the right tympanic membrane. The scutum ('shield') is a thin plate of bone that obscures the view of the heads of the malleus and incus. It may be eroded by cholesteatoma and hence this area must always be inspected.

RINNE AND WEBER TUNING FORK TESTING

Although there have been various reports regarding the reliability of tuning fork tests (1), they are simple, quick and invaluable aids in the diagnosis of hearing loss (2). Tuning fork tests can be used to confirm audiometric findings, especially if the hearing test does not seem to be congruent with the clinical findings. They are also useful as a quick bedside test for checking that the patient has not suffered a dead ear following surgery.

Traditionally, a 512 Hz tuning fork is used for testing. Low-frequency tuning forks provide greater vibrotactile stimulation (which can be misinterpreted as an audible signal by the patient), while high-frequency tuning forks have a higher rate of decay (i.e. the tone does not last long after the tuning fork has been struck). There is evidence to suggest, however, that a 256 Hz tuning fork is more reliable than a 512 Hz tuning fork (3, 4).

The commonest tuning fork tests performed are the Rinne's and Weber's tests. They must be performed in conjunction in order to diagnose a conductive or sensorineural hearing loss.

Rinne's test

A 512 Hz tuning fork is struck on the elbow. It is essential that the examiner checks that they can hear the tuning fork as this also serves as a comparative test of hearing. The tuning fork is presented to the patient with the prongs of the fork held vertically and in line with the ear canal. The patient is asked if they can hear a sound. The tuning fork is held by the ear for a few moments before its base is firmly pressed against the mastoid process behind the ear. The patient is asked, 'Is it louder in front or when I place it on your head?'

As air conduction (AC) is better than bone conduction (BC) in a normal hearing ear, the tuning fork is heard louder in front of the ear than when placed behind the ear (i.e. AC > BC). This is described as Rinne +ve; if bone conduction is greater than air conduction, this is Rinne −ve.

Weber's test

A 512 Hz tuning fork is struck on the elbow and firmly placed on the patient's forehead. The patient is asked, 'Is the sound louder in your left ear, right ear, or somewhere in the middle?'

As the hearing in both ears should be the same, in a normal subject the sound heard will be 'in the middle'.

Interpretation

In order to diagnose a conductive or sensorineural hearing loss, both Rinne's and Weber's tests must be performed (Figure 2.3).

If Rinne's test is +ve on the left and −ve on the right, and Weber's test lateralizes to the right side, this suggests a conductive hearing loss in the right ear.

If Rinne's test is −ve on the right and +ve on the left, and Weber's test lateralizes to the left side, this suggests a right sensorineural hearing loss in the right ear.

Anterior rhinoscopy

The head mirror is often approached with some trepidation by the junior ENT surgeon, who may feel self-conscious as the mirror can be cumbersome. Many departments use headlights as an alternative.

A right-handed examiner should position the Bull's lamp over the patient's left shoulder at head height and wear the head mirror over their right eye. The lamp light can be directed onto the head mirror and the beam focused onto the patient.

Examine the profile of the nose, looking for external deviation of the nasal dorsum. Check for bruising, swelling, signs of infection, nasal discharge and scars.

Gently raise the tip of the nose to allow you to examine the vestibule of the nose and the anteroinferior end of the nasal septum.

The Thudichum speculum is held in the nondominant hand (i.e. the left if the examiner is right-handed), leaving the dominant hand free to use any instruments.

Hold the metal loop on your index finger with the finger pointing towards you and the prongs away from you.

Swing your middle finger to one side of the Thudichum and your ring finger to the other. You can now squeeze the Thudichum and use the prongs to open the nares to examine the nasal cavity. This provides a view of the nasal septum, inferior turbinate and head of the middle turbinate. A flexible nasolaryngoscope or a rigid endoscope is required in order to assess the middle meatus, posterior nasal cavity and postnasal space.

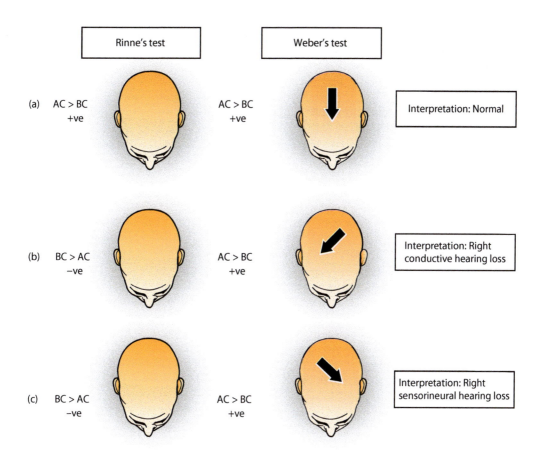

Rinne's test		Weber's test	
(a) AC > BC +ve	AC > BC +ve		Interpretation: Normal
(b) BC > AC −ve	AC > BC +ve		Interpretation: Right conductive hearing loss
(c) BC > AC −ve	AC > BC +ve		Interpretation: Right sensorineural hearing loss

Figure 2.3. Interpretation of tuning fork tests.

In children, especially if a foreign body is suspected, it is often kinder simply to lift the tip of the nose rather than use a Thudichum speculum. Alternatively, an otoscope provides an excellent view.

Nasal patency is assessed by placing a metal speculum under the nose. Misting or condensation on the metal surface during expiration provides a measure of nasal patency.

▌ Ear microsuction

Explain to the patient that microsuction is required in order to remove debris and wax from the external auditory canal. Warn the patient that they will hear a loud hissing noise and may experience temporary dizziness following the procedure.

Position the patient supine (or sitting in a chair) with the head turned to the opposite side. With the microscope illuminating the ear, take this opportunity to study the pinna, canal opening and surrounding skin for scars or sinuses.

Adjust the eye pieces and start with the lowest magnification. Use the largest speculum that will comfortably enter the external auditory canal. Hold the speculum between the index finger and thumb, place the middle finger into the conchal bowl and gently pull the pinna posteriorly. This will open and straighten the ear canal. If the ear canal is narrow, use a smaller speculum or ask the patient to open their mouth (this manoeuvre often increases the anteroposterior diameter of the canal as the condyle of the mandible is related to the anterior canal wall).

Assess the canal wall and contents. Remember that the hairy outer third of the canal is relatively insensitive but the thin inner skin is extremely sensitive. Any contact with the speculum or suction will produce a great deal of discomfort.

Using a wide bore sucker, begin by removing debris within the lateral hairy portion of the canal. Aim to touch only the debris and not the canal skin. Try to remove all the debris, especially in cases of otitis externa where debris will result in an ongoing infection if not removed. A wax hook may be used as an alternative method for wax removal.

If the debris or wax is too hard or the procedure too uncomfortable for the patient, a course of sodium bicarbonate ear drops (two drops three times a day for two weeks) will be required before a further attempt at wax removal is made.

If the tympanic membrane is obscured, microsuction along the anterior canal wall until the tympanic membrane is visible (the tympanic membrane is continuous with the posterior canal wall and can be damaged if microsuction follows the posterior canal wall).

If there is trauma to the ear canal or if bleeding occurs, prescribe a short course of antibiotic ear drops, warning the patient of the risk of ototoxicity.

▌ Flexible nasolaryngoscopy

Explain the procedure to the patient and ask the patient which side of their nose is the easier to breathe through, selecting this side for examination. Spray the chosen side with local anaesthetic or insert a cotton wool pledget soaked in local anaesthetic. Patients often describe numbness of the upper lip or back of their tongue,

which can be used as a guide to the level of anaesthesia.

The nasoendoscope may be used with or without a sheath, depending on local decontamination protocols. Clean the tip of the scope with an alcohol wipe to prevent condensation and apply a thin film of lubricant gel to the distal 5 cm of the nasoendoscope. Ensure the gel does not cover the tip of the scope as this will occlude your view. The patient's saliva provides an effective alternative.

Ask the patient to breathe through their mouth and, holding the end of the scope between the index finger and thumb, place the tip of the nasoendoscope into the nasal cavity. Ensure full control of the scope by placing the middle finger on the tip of the patient's nose. If a patient were to fall forward, the nasoendoscope will not be driven into the nasal cavity.

Insert the scope into the nostril and pass it along the floor of the nose with the inferior turbinate laterally and septum medially. Posteriorly, the Eustachian tube orifice and postnasal space will come into view (see Chapter 1, Figure 1.2). If the septum is deviated and the scope cannot be easily advanced, try to pass it between the inferior and middle turbinates (laterally) and the septum (medially). If this is too uncomfortable for the patient, the other nasal cavity may be used.

With the postnasal space in view, ask the patient to breathe in through their nose. This opens the inlet into the oropharynx. Use the control toggle to flex the distal end of the scope inferiorly and gently advance.

The uvula and soft palate will slide away and the base of tongue and larynx will come into view (see Chapter 1, Figure 1.14).

Adopt a system to ensure that all aspects of this region are examined. The following is a guide: tongue base, valleculae, epiglottis (lingual and laryngeal surfaces), supraglottis, interarytenoid bar, vocal cords (appearance and mobility), subglottis, pyriform fossae and posterior pharyngeal wall. The larynx may be difficult to view in those patients with an infantile epiglottis or prominent tongue base. Where this is encountered, ask the patient to point their chin up to the ceiling to draw the tongue base forward and bring the larynx into view. To assess the pyriform fossae, ask the patient to blow their cheeks out while you pinch their nose. If secretions obscure your view, ask the patient to swallow.

Remove the scope gently and supply patients with tissues to use after completing the examination.

▌ Rigid nasoendoscopy

Rigid endoscopy of the nasal cavity requires a systematic examination involving three passes with either a 0° or 30° scope (Figure 2.4).

Figure 2.4. Rigid endoscopy. The first pass of the endoscope should pass along the floor of the nose, the second into the middle meatus and the third into the superior meatus and olfactory niche.

The first pass provides an overall view of the anterior nasal cavity, the septum and the floor of the nasal cavity to the posterior choana. The Eustachian tube cushion, orifice and the fossa of Rosenmüller and adenoidal pad must also be examined.

The second is into the middle meatus and allows identification of the uncinate process, middle meatal ostium and ethmoidal bulla. The third examines the superior meatus and olfactory niche; the sphenoid ostium may be identified during this pass.

▌ Examination of the oral cavity

Ensure that both you and the patient are seated comfortably, at the same level.

Using the head mirror or headlight, begin by examining the lips and face of the patient. Note any scars or petechiae.

It is important to be systematic (Figure 2.5).

Use two tongue depressors. Begin by asking the patient to open their mouth and insert one tongue depressor onto the buccal surface of each cheek and ask the patient to clench their teeth. Gently pulling laterally, withdraw the blades examining the buccal mucosa, gingivae, teeth, parotid duct orifices and buccal sulci. Anteriorly, draw the blades superiorly to examine beneath the upper lip and repeat with the lower lip.

Ask the patient to open their mouth and study the superior surface of the tongue. With the

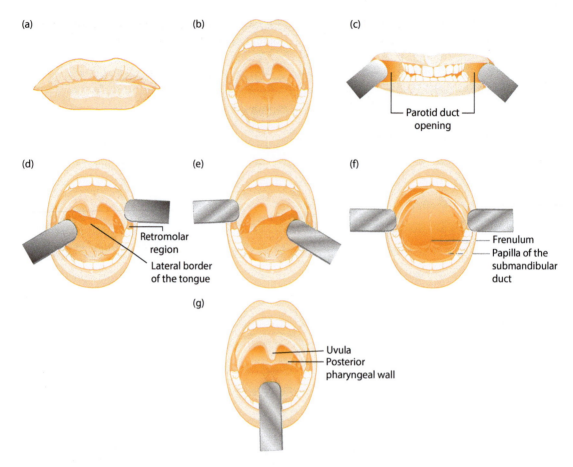

(a)

(b)

(c) Parotid duct opening

(d) Retromolar region / Lateral border of the tongue

(e)

(f) Frenulum / Papilla of the submandibular duct

(g) Uvula / Posterior pharyngeal wall

Figure 2.5. Examination of the oral cavity. A systematic approach must be used to assess the oral cavity fully.

tongue pointing superiorly, examine the floor of the mouth and inferior surface of the tongue. The openings of the submandibular ducts are found just lateral to the frenulum of the tongue.

Using both tongue blades again, examine the retromolar regions and lateral borders of the tongue.

Ask the patient to keep their tongue in their mouth and keep breathing. Gently depress the anterior half of the tongue, avoiding the posterior third as this can make patients gag. Examine both tonsils, comparing their relative size. Inspect the oropharynx, including uvula and movements of

the soft palate. Ask the patient to look up to the ceiling and examine the hard palate.

Palpate the tongue including the tongue base. Submucosal tumours in these structures can often be palpated before they are seen. Where the history is suggestive of an abnormality of the submandibular gland or duct, bimanual palpation should be used.

▌ Examination of the neck and facial nerve function

Inspect the general appearance of the patient, noting any facial scars or asymmetry of facial tone at rest. Ensure adequate exposure of the patient by removing neck ties and unfasten the upper shirt buttons so that both clavicles are visualized.

Inspect the neck, noting scars, sinuses, masses or tattoos (these were previously used to mark radiotherapy fields).

Stand behind the subject and sequentially palpate the same lymph node levels on both sides of the neck simultaneously (Figure 2.5). It is important to be systematic. Start with the submental then submandibular triangles (level 1), followed by the jugulodigastric and jugular lymph nodes (levels 2, 3, 4) by palpating along the anterior border of each sternocleidomastoid muscle and the paratracheal region. Examine the posterior triangle nodes. Working posteriorly, palpate the parotid gland and postaural and occipital lymph nodes.

Once again, palpate the laryngeal skeleton and thyroid gland from behind. Note the site, size and appearance of any mass and whether it is tethered to the skin or underlying muscles. Assess whether the mass moves with swallowing (give the patient a glass of water to drink) or tongue protrusion. Auscultate for a bruit and, in the case of a thyroid mass with retrosternal extension, percuss from superior to inferior along the sternum.

▌ Examination of facial nerve function

Sitting level with the patient, examine their general appearance and for any scars or masses.

Ask the patient to raise their eyebrows and compare both sides. Remember that there is crossover in the innervation of this region so that a patient is still able to wrinkle their forehead in a unilateral upper motor neuron palsy.

Ask the patient to shut their eyes tightly, flare their nostrils, blow out their cheeks and bare their teeth. Where facial weakness is observed, blinking repeatedly may reveal synkinesis where reinnervation has occurred along incorrect pathways; contraction of obicularis oris muscle may result in contraction of the angle of the mouth.

All patients must have their facial weakness graded so that any changes can be monitored.

The most commonly used grading system is the House–Brackmann facial nerve grading system. Note that there is complete eye closure in a grade 3 and incomplete eye closure in a grade 4 facial palsy.

Grade 1 – Normal.
Grade 2 – Slight weakness with good eye closure with minimal effort, good forehead movement and slight asymmetry of the mouth.
Grade 3 – Symmetry and normal tone at rest with obvious weakness, although complete eye closure and asymmetrical mouth movement with effort.
Grade 4 – Incomplete eye closure, no movement of the forehead, but symmetry and normal tone at rest.
Grade 5 – Asymmetry at rest with barely perceptible movement of the mouth and incomplete eye closure.
Grade 6 – No movement.

When faced with a true lower motor neuron palsy, look for a cause by examining the remaining cranial nerves, perform otoscopy to exclude middle ear pathology and palpate the parotid glands. Audiology is required with tympanometry, a pure tone audiogram and, occasionally, stapedial reflexes.

REFERENCES

1 Burkey JM, Lippy WH, Schuring AG, Rizer FM. 1998. Clinical utility of the 512-Hz Rinne tuning fork test. *Am J Otol* 19: 59–62.
2 Behn A, Westerberg BD, Zhang H et al. 2007. Accuracy of the Weber and Rinne tuning fork tests in evaluation of children with otitis media with effusion. *J Otolaryngol* 36: 197–202.
3 Browning GG, Swan IR. 1988. Sensitivity and specificity of Rinne tuning fork test. *BMJ* 297: 1381–2.
4 Browning GG, Swan IR, Chew KK. 1989. Clinical role of informal tests of hearing. *J Laryngol Otol* 103: 7–11.

3 COMMON ENT PATHOLOGY

Ketan Desai

OTITIS EXTERNA

Otitis externa is inflammation of the external auditory canal. It is common, extremely painful and often precipitated by irritants such as cotton buds. There may be an infective component, commonly bacterial, such as *Pseudomonas aeruginosa*, *Staphylococcus aureus* and *Proteus*, or less frequently fungal, such as *Aspergillus* species or *Candida albicans*. The external auditory canal is often swollen and filled with debris that requires microsuction. Treatment generally consists of one week of ear drops containing a combination of steroid and antibiotic. Fungal infections require a 3–4-week course of anti-fungal drops. An ear swab is useful in directing antibiotic selection where the infection does not resolve with the initial treatment.

When the external ear canal is very swollen, a wick is inserted to splint the meatus open to allow penetration of the topical treatment. This should be removed as the swelling decreases, usually after 48 hours. The infection may progress to involve the pinna and peri-auricular soft tissues (cellulitis), necessitating hospital admission for intravenous antibiotics. Sometimes the infection is localized and a small abscess, or furuncle can form. This is commonly caused by *S. aureus* infection of a hair follicle in the ear canal and is extremely painful. Incision and drainage are often required, together with topical antibiotics.

An important differential diagnosis of otitis externa is malignant otitis externa. This is an osteomyelitis of the ear canal and lateral skull base, which occurs more frequently in diabetics and immunocompromised patients presenting with severe pain. *Pseudomonas aeruginosa* is the most common cause and the typical otoscopic appearance is granulation tissue or exposed bone on the floor of the ear canal. As the infection spreads through the skull base, the lower cranial nerves (CN VII–XII) are affected. MRI is useful in determining the extent of the disease, although it lags behind clinical signs of improvement with treatment. Treatment is a prolonged course of intravenous antibiotics followed by further oral antibiotics (twelve week), regular microsuction, topical antibiotic–steroid ear drops, good glycaemic control and analgesia. A biopsy is often needed to exclude malignancy and determine microbiological sensitivities. Radioisotope scans (e.g. gallium) or magnetic resonance imaging (MRI) can be used to assess the response to treatment.

IMPACTED WAX

Ear wax is composed of secretions from sebaceous and apocrine glands in the lateral third of the ear canal mixed with dead squamous cells. It becomes impacted in 10% of children, 5% of healthy adults and nearly 60% of the elderly (1). Although often asymptomatic, it may cause a conductive hearing loss and discomfort. Impacted wax needs to be removed to facilitate examination of the tympanic membrane. In primary care, removal is facilitated by the use of ceruminolytic agents (2) or ear syringing. Syringing is, however, contraindicated in those who have a tympanic membrane perforation or who have developed otitis externa from previous syringing. In otolaryngology departments wax is removed under the microscope using a Zoellner sucker, wax hook, Jobson–Horne probe or crocodile forceps. Care should be taken to avoid trauma to the ear canal. The use of cotton buds by the patient should be discouraged as this impacts wax and traumatises the ear canal causing otitis externa.

ACUTE OTITIS MEDIA (AOM)

Inflammation of middle ear mucosa mainly affects young children as part of an upper respiratory tract infection. Causative organisms include viruses and bacteria, such as *Streptococcus pneumoniae, Haemophilus influenzae* and *Moraxella catarrhalis*. Patients present with general symptoms of irritability, pyrexia and nausea, with ENT symptoms of otalgia and hearing loss. Examination reveals a bulging erythematous tympanic membrane, which may perforate and discharge pus. Initial treatment is supportive, with simple analgesia or antipyretics. If symptoms persist, oral antibiotics such as amoxicillin or clarithromycin are indicated (3). Frequent episodes of AOM (more than four episodes over six months) require ENT referral. Recurrent otitis media may be treated by insertion of grommets or a prolonged course of low dose antibiotics.

Rare but potentially serious complications of AOM (and more commonly of acute mastoiditis – see below) can be classified anatomically into three groups:

1 Intratemporal – Tympanic membrane perforation, facial nerve palsy (particularly if the tympanic segment of facial nerve is dehiscent) and acute mastoiditis with mastoid abscess.
2 Intracranial – Meningitis, brain abscess, encephalitis and sigmoid sinus thrombosis.
3 Systemic – Septicaemia, septic arthritis and endocarditis.

OTITIS MEDIA WITH EFFUSION (OME) (GLUE EAR)

Persistent otitis media with bilateral effusions (OME) is the most common cause of hearing loss in children. The typical audiological finding is a mild to moderate conductive hearing loss, associated with a flat (type B) tympanogram. Bilateral grommet insertion is indicated (4) where effusions persist for over three months associated with a hearing level in the better hearing ear of 25–30 dB HL or worse, averaged at 0.5, 1, 2 and 4 kHz.

Children with Down's syndrome should be offered hearing aids rather than grommet surgery if they have OME. Children with cleft palate can be offered grommets as an alternative to hearing aids.

Adults with persistent unilateral OME should undergo a examination of the postnasal space under general anaesthesia, with a biopsy taken from the fossa of Rosenmüller, immediately posterior to the Eustachian tube orifice, to exclude the possibility of a nasopharyngeal tumour.

ACUTE MASTOIDITIS

Acute mastoiditis is an inflammatory process affecting the mastoid air cells; it occurs most commonly in children. It is an uncommon complication of AOM. Patients are generally unwell, with spiking temperatures. There is a postauricular abscess with lateral and anterior displacement of the pinna and tenderness over the mastoid bone. Early cases may respond to medical treatment with intravenous antibiotics, analgesia and hydration (5). A contrast-enhanced CT scan is used to exclude a brain abscess, lateral sinus thrombosis, and assess temporal bone anatomy. If there is failure to improve, where there is an established postaural abscess, or if the suspicion of complications demands surgical intervention a cortical mastoidectomy and grommet insertion with placement of a corrugated drain within the postauricular wound is undertaken.

PINNA HAEMATOMA

Blunt trauma to the pinna may result in a subperichondrial haematoma. Since the cartilage gains its nutrient supply from the overlying perichondrium, an untreated pinna haematoma results in cartilage necrosis and permanent deformity – 'cauliflower ear'. Needle aspiration of a pinna haematoma followed by a compression bandage is rarely effective. A small incision through the overlying skin under local anaesthetic allows continued drainage and is a more definitive treatment (6). The incision should be placed where the scar will be least visible, ideally along the rim of the conchal bowl, under the helical rim or approached from the cranial surface of the pinna (with a small window of cartilage excised). Through-and-through sutures can be placed to secure silastic splints or dental rolls, to achieve more reliable pressure and to prevent haematoma recurrence under the head bandage. All patients should receive co-amoxiclav or an equivalent antibiotic to prevent perichondritis and should be reviewed after 7 days for suture removal.

PERICHONDRITIS AND PINNA CELLULITIS

Inflammation of the perichondrium (perichondritis) can result in permanent deformity of the pinna. It commonly occurs as a result of bacterial infection following trauma to the pinna from piercing, insect bite or skin abrasion, although can also be secondary to otitis externa.

The pinna is swollen, erythematous and extremely tender. Previous episodes of perichondritis or inflammation of other cartilaginous structures should be looked into in order to exclude relapsing perichondritis.

Perichondritis and pinna cellulitis require a combination of intravenous and oral antibiotics as cartilage compromise can lead to marked disfigurement of the pinna. Piercings in the affected ear should be removed. Rarely, surgery is required to drain a collection or debride necrotic soft tissue (7).

SUDDEN SENSORINEURAL HEARING LOSS (SSHL)

This is a unilateral or bilateral subjective deterioration in hearing, which develops over seconds to hours and on objective testing is confirmed to be sensorineural in nature.

A conductive hearing loss should first be excluded by careful examination of the ear, tuning fork tests and a pure tone audiogram. In 88% of cases, no obvious cause is found, but a careful history and examination should consider potential infective, autoimmune, vascular, traumatic, neoplastic and neurological causes (8). Competing theories for idiopathic cases include viral and vascular insults to the inner ear and rupture of the cochlear membrane. Approximately 60% of patients improve with or without intervention. Standard treatment is with prednisolone (oral for one week first line and or injected into the middle ear if there is no imporvement) (9). There is poor evidence for efficacy with aspirin, betahistine (10), acyclovir and inhaled carbogen (oxygen mixed with 5% CO_2) (11). Unilateral loss may be managed in the outpatient setting, but those with bilateral loss require admission for investigation (blood tests to exclude autoimmune causes and MRI scanning).

FACIAL NERVE PALSY

There are a wide variety of causes for a facial nerve palsy. Lower motor neurone lesions are distinguished from upper motor neurone lesions by the absence of forehead movement (forehead movement is spared in upper motor neurone lesions as a result of the bilateral upper motor neurone distribution supplying this area). All patients must have their degree of facial weakness recorded using the House–Brackmann scale.

Lower motor neurone pathology can occur anywhere along the path of the affected nerve. An assessment of the cranial nerves, ear, parotid gland, oral cavity and neck examination is mandatory.

Causes include Bell's palsy, Ramsay Hunt Syndrome, malignant otits externa, ear or parotid surgery, middle ear disease, temporal bone fracture and iatrogenic trauma.

▌ Bells palsy

This syndrome of facial paralysis is a diagnosis of exclusion. Although described as idiopathic, there is evidence to suggest that the palsy occurs due to herpes reactivation. A thorough history and examination are required. An MRI is only indicated if this is a recurrent palsy or if the palsy fails to recover (12).

Initial treatment is with oral prednisolone (1 mg per kg, typically 60 mg for an adult) for seven days.

Although there is inconclusive evidence to support the use of antivirals, acyclovir (800 mg five times a day for 10 days) is also often prescribed (13) along with one week of oral prednisolone. Any patient with a facial nerve palsy who is unable to close their eye (House–Brackmann grade 4–6) must use artificial tears and tape their eyes closed at night in order to protect the cornea. If the eye becomes painful or red, an urgent ophthalmic opinion should be sought.

Approximately 60% of patients with an idiopathic palsy recover to House–Brackmann grade 1 or 2. A further 12% suffer a recurrence on the same or contralateral side.

▌ Ramsay Hunt syndrome

This condition is caused by herpes zoster. The facial palsy is accompanied by painful vesicles on the pinna or external auditory canal, and occasionally the soft palate. The onset is rapid, and the 8th nerve may become involved with concurrent hearing loss and vertigo.

Treatment is similar to that of Bell's palsy (14, 15).

▌ Acute suppurative otitis media (ASOM)

An acute otitis media may result in a facial nerve palsy, typically if the bony canal of the facial nerve is dehiscent within the middle ear cleft. Treatment includes intravenous antibiotics, oral steroids and CT of the temporal bone may be of value in order to exclude chronic suppurative otitis media (CSOM). A myringotomy may be considered appropriate if there is no clinical improvement following 24–48 hours of medical treatment.

FOREIGN BODIES – EAR

Foreign bodies within the external ear canal commonly affect children and may be difficult to remove. Children will need to be held by a parent or nurse, and the first attempt at removal is often the only chance. If the foreign body cannot be removed, a short general anaesthetic in the following few days is indicated to allow removal. The exception are batteries, which are corrosive and must be removed that day. Objects can be removed under the microscope using wax hook, microsuction or irrigation (Figure 3.1). The use of crocodile forceps can result in medial displacement of the foreign bodies and their use should be restricted to objects that can be grasped. Insects should be drowned using olive oil prior to removal. *Do not* attempt to flush out tablets, seeds or nuts (organic materials) as these swell and become more difficult to remove.

∎ Trauma

Every patient undergoing middle ear surgery must have their facial nerve function recorded pre- and post-operatively. Iatrogenic damage requires surgical reexploration and nerve repair.

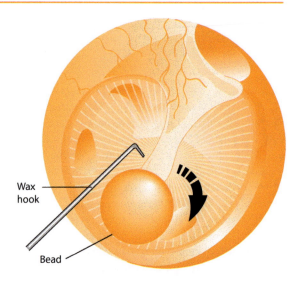

Wax hook

Bead

Figure 3.1. Removal of a bead from the external auditory canal.

TYMPANIC MEMBRANE TRAUMA

Pressure changes or direct trauma can damage the external auditory canal and tympanic membrane. On otoscopy, the tympanic membrane is often obscured by blood. Tuning fork tests and audiograms are used to assess hearing. Hearing loss may be conductive due to blood in the middle or external ear or ossicular discontinuity. Sensorineural hearing loss is more common when there is an accompanying temporal bone fracture.

Treatment is generally conservative. Patients are reassured and advised to keep their ear dry and have an outpatient follow-up at six weeks, where spontaneous healing of tympanic membrane is usually confirmed. An audiogram documents return of hearing to normal.

TEMPORAL BONE FRACTURES

The temporal bone contains many vital structures, including the facial nerve, cochlea, labyrinth, ossicles, internal carotid artery, jugular vein and sigmoid sinus. Temporal bone fractures are traditionally classified as longitudinal, transverse and oblique in relation to the petrous ridge of the temporal bone. The usefulness of this classification system has been questioned and a newer system of categorizing injuries on CT as oticcapsule violating and oticcapsule sparing, has been shown to be more predictive of complications (16). Initially, advanced trauma life support (ATLS) management takes priority as temporal bone fractures can be associated with significant head injury. Clinical signs include blood in the ear canal, haemotympanum and Battle's sign (postauricular bruising). Of more concern are sensorineural hearing loss, vertigo, facial nerve injury and cerebral spinal fluid (CSF) otorrhoea.

Facial nerve function immediately after injury must be documented. CT scanning is helpful in excluding intracranial injury, identifying damage to important intratemporal structures and classifying the type of fracture. Immediate onset severe facial nerve paralysis is suggestive of nerve transection and may require surgical exploration. However, most traumatic facial nerve palsies are delayed in onset, secondary to fracture-related nerve oedema and are treated conservatively with steroids.

FOREIGN BODIES – NOSE

Foreign bodies in the nose should be removed as soon as possible as there is a theoretical risk of aspiration (Figure 3.2). As with foreign bodies in the ear, children need to be held by a parent or nurse, often with a blanket wrapped around the body and arms. A headlight, suction and wax hook allow removal in most cases. A useful additional removal technique is the 'parent's kiss', whereby the parent blows air into the mouth of the child while occluding the contralateral nostril (17). If these manoeuvres are unsuccessful, a short general anaesthetic is required for removal.

Wax hook

Figure 3.2. Removal of a foreign body from the nasal cavity.

NASAL TRAUMA

Nasal trauma may result in a deviated nasal bridge. A patient who has sustained nasal injury, with suspected deviation of the nasal bones should first be assessed for other injuries (ATLS protocol).

The nose should be examined to exclude a septal haematoma and any epistaxis managed. Swelling over the nose may prevent an accurate assessment of the position of the nasal bones. Hence, the patient should be recalled 5–7 days post injury and the nasal bridge reassessed.

If the nasal bones are deviated, and the patient desires it, the nose can be manipulated under local or general anaesthesia (18). It is essential that this is performed within 14 days of the initial injury as the bridge may become fixed, making simple manipulation impossible. Risks include epistaxis, periorbital bruising and septal haematoma. Patients should be warned that the aim is to straighten the bony bridge and that their nose may appear different after the injury. The nose will remain unstable until the bones have rehealed and so further injury should be avoided.

SEPTAL HAEMATOMA/ABSCESS

Septal haematomas can rapidly develop following nasal trauma or after septal surgery. A haematoma can become secondarily infected, resulting in an abscess. Patients describe nasal obstruction and pain. Examination usually reveals bilateral septal swelling, which is compressible on palpation. Pus may be seen lying on the surface of the septum.

Patients require formal incision and drainage under general anaesthetic. A hemitransfixion incision is made and a corrugated drain sutured in place (a trouser drain may be required with a 'leg' on either side of the septal cartilage). Antibiotic treatment is required following abscess drainage and a pus swab sent to microbiology. A septal haematoma or abscess should be seen within a few hours and operated on within a day, as prolonged devascularisation of the cartilage results in its reabsorption resulting in nasal deformity (19). In addition, infection may extend intracranially via the ophthalmic veins to involve the cavernous sinus.

ACUTE SINUSITIS

Acute sinusitis is generally managed in primary care with oral antibiotics and nasal decongestants. It commonly occurs following an acute upper respiratory tract infection and presents with purulent nasal discharge, nasal obstruction and facial pain that is worse on bending forward.

Patients may be referred if there are concerns regarding complications of sinusitis such as periorbital cellulitis. Fungal sinusitis should be considered when assessing patients who are immunocompromised.

PERIORBITAL CELLULITIS

Periorbital cellulitis is an ENT emergency and patients may become blind within a matter of hours. A subperiosteal abscess may arise due to spread of infection from the ethmoidal air cells laterally into the orbital cavity. Patients often describe a recent upper respiratory tract infection.

These patients must be discussed promptly with a senior colleague so that they can be reviewed or their management discussed.

The eyelid may be swollen with associated chemosis, and there may be proptosis of the eye. It is important to assess red colour vision, in particular, and this may be performed using an Ishihara chart. Visual acuity and eye movements also require regular monitoring. Restricted eye movement or pain on eye movement is often associated with an abscess.

Given that the condition predominantly occurs in children, such an examination can be challenging and it is worth seeking paediatric and ophthalmological consultations early. Patients with periorbital cellulitis or a potential intraorbital collection should be discussed promptly with a senior so that they can be reviewed or their management discussed.

An urgent CT scan of the paranasal sinuses is essential. For young children preparations may be made to perform the scan under general anaesthetic, proceeding to surgery if the imaging reveals a collection. Children should receive appropriate analgesia, intravenous antibiotics (normally a third generation cephalosporin) and, if there is evidence of sinusitis, paediatric nasal decongestant.

Surgical decompression of a subperiosteal abscess is performed endoscopically or via a Lynch–Howarth incision. A drain is required if an open approach is used.

TONSILLITIS

Tonsillitis is most commonly bacterial, caused by *Streptococci, Staphylococci* or *Haemophilus influenzae*. Viral infections also occur, most commonly the *Epstein–Barr* virus (EBV), which is the cause of infectious mononucleosis or glandular fever. Patients have a painful throat with odynophagia (pain on swallowing) and sometimes referred otalgia. They are treated in primary care with phenoxymethylpenicillin (Penicillin V), or a macrolide if they are penicillin-allergic. Ampicillin, Amoxicillin and Co-Amoxiclav should be avoided as these can precipitate a severe scarring rash in patients with EBV and the patient being incorrectly labeled as penicillin allergic.

If patients are unable to swallow fluids, they should be admitted to hospital for rehydration and intravenous antibiotics. Blood samples are sent for a full blood count, electrolytes, liver function tests, C-reactive protein and the locally-agreed test for EBV.

Intravenous benzylpenicillin is required, and oral soluble paracetamol, codeine and a non-steroidal anti-inflammatory for analgesia. Tonsillar enlargement may cause airway obstruction, and if there is any suggestion of compromise, patients must undergo flexible nasolaryngoscopy. In such cases, these patients should be given steroids (either 8 mg dexamethasone IV or hydrocortisone 200 mg IV), discussed with a senior colleague and closely monitored in an ENT airway observation bed or in a high dependency or critical care unit. If, conversely, a patient complains of a severe sore throat and has tonsils with *normal* appearances, immediate nasolaryngoscopy should be performed to assess whether the diagnosis is supraglottitis.

Inpatient treatment is normally required for no more than 24–48 hours, and patients are discharged with analgesia and oral antibiotics. A short course of steroids may be useful in patients with glandular fever, and they should also be advised to refrain from alcohol for two months while their liver recovers from the acute injury. They should also be advised to avoid contact sport as EBV-induced hepatosplenomegaly can put them at risk of internal bleeding from abdominal injury. If patients meet the criteria for tonsillectomy (see *tonsillectomy* section) this can be considered after the inflammation has settled – an 'interval' tonsillectomy.

PERITONSILLAR ABSCESS

Also known as a quinsy, a peritonsillar abscess is a collection of pus that develops between the tonsillar capsule and the surrounding superior constrictor muscle. This condition mainly occurs in young adults, as a result of acute tonsillitis.

On examination, the patient has trismus (an inability to fully open the mouth), and the uvula is pushed away from the midline by swelling under the soft palate. If large, a quinsy may cause airway compromise.

The soft palate is first sprayed with local anaesthetic, and the collection aspirated to confirm the presence of pus. A 19G white needle on a luer-lock and 10 or 20 mL syringe is used (1 cm of the tip of the needle sheath can be cut off and the remainder of the sheath replaced on the needle to act as a guard preventing over-insertion). The needle is pointed towards the back of the mouth (rather than drifting laterally), and the area of maximal fluctuance aspirated (or on an arc between a third of the way, and half way from the base of the uvula to the last upper molar).

Incision and drainage can be performed in the same location using a no.11 blade with tape wrapped around the blade to expose only the distal 1 cm.

The incision can be opened by the use of Tilley's dressing forceps, and a Yankauer sucker can be used to remove the purulent material.

Patients are usually admitted and treated as for severe tonsillitis with intravenous antibiotics, although where symptoms completely resolve after drainage, outpatient antibiotic therapy may be sufficient. It is helpful to send a sample to microbiology to guide antibiotic therapy, although patients are usually managed with benzylpenicillin and metronidazole. If the abscess recollects, or there is neck swelling, a parapharyngeal abscess should be suspected and a CT scan performed to investigate this.

SUPRAGLOTTITIS

Supraglottitis is inflammation of the soft tissues immediately above the vocal cords. It is normally caused by *Haemophilus influenzae*, *Streptococcus pneumoniae* or *S. pyogenes*. Patients usually complain of a short history of a sore throat with rapid hoarseness and dysphagia. This may be sufficiently severe to prevent them from swallowing their saliva.

These patients must be assessed as a priority as the airway can rapidly deteriorate. Shortness of breath, tachypnoea or stridor are worrying features and a senior ENT and anaesthetic input should always be sought. Flexible nasolaryngoscopy should be performed with caution where significant airway obstruction is present. Depending on the severity of the airway compromise patients may be nursed in ITU or a high dependency unit, but the milder cases may be observed in an easily-visible 'airway' bed on an ENT ward.

Adrenaline nebulisers (1 mL of 1:1000, or diluted in 4 mL of normal saline) are effective in reducing some of the mucosal swelling. Heliox (Helium/oxygen) provides relief as this low density gas increases flow. Patients should be cannulated and given intravenous dexamethasone 8 mg or hydrocortisone 200 mg to help reduce mucosal oedema, although this only works fully after a few hours. Intravenous third generation cephalosporins are normally the antibiotic of choice. These patients may need intervention to secure their airway such as intubation, or emergency cricothyroidotomy prior to a formal tracheostomy.

EPIGLOTTITIS

Severe inflammation of the epiglottis in children is fortunately now rare as a result of the *Haemophilus influenzae* Type B vaccine (20, 21).

Children present with stridor; drooling is common, and 'sitting upright' (in the 'sniffing the morning air' position) to maximize the available airway.

Any potential stimulant can send them into complete airway obstruction. These children should neither be examined nor cannulated. A senior anaesthetist and ENT surgeon must be called. The patient is taken to theatre in order to secure the airway by intubation, although an emergency tracheostomy may occasionally be required. Patients are kept intubated and treated with intravenous antibiotics until a leak around the cuff of the endotracheal tube is observed, an indication of decreased airway swelling.

SMOKE INHALATION

Patients who have been exposed to dense smoke are often admitted under chest physicians. The upper airway must not be neglected. The effects of smoke injury on the larynx can develop over several hours and these patients should be closely monitored in hospital in a high dependency setting. Singeing of the nasal hair, soot in the nasal cavity or passages or oral mucosa, and voice change indicate smoke inhalation.

Nasolaryngoscopy should be performed to visualize the larynx and this may need to be repeated if symptoms deteriorate. Steroids can be useful in reducing mucosal oedema. These patients should be discussed with a senior promptly, because development of marked laryngeal inflammation may prevent intubation and necessitate a tracheostomy to secure the airway.

PARAPHARYNGEAL ABSCESS

An abscess may form within the parapharyngeal space. This is an inverted pyramidal space bounded superiorly by the skull base, medially by the pharynx, posteriorly by the prevertebral muscles, laterally by the mandible and parotid fascia, with its apex at the greater cornu of the hyoid bone.

Infection may arise from a dental or pharyngeal source (commonly tonsil). The carotid sheath runs through the parapharyngeal space and therefore infections in this area can lead to thrombosis of the great vessels or airway compromise (22). Patients report throat discomfort and unilateral neck swelling, with limitation of movement, and may have trismus. There will be a palpable swelling in the upper neck near the angle of the jaw, with medialisation of the oropharynx. History and examination findings should help identify the initial source of the infection and antibiotics (normally a cephalosporin and metronidazole) should be commenced intravenously. Patients require a contrast-enhanced CT scan to confirm the presence of a collection and to plan potential surgical drainage (these include an external neck approach, or via a trans-oral route following excision of the tonsil). Patients should, therefore, remain starved until discussed with a senior colleague.

RETROPHARYNGEAL ABSCESS

In the absence of a penetrating foreign body, a retropharyngeal abscess normally occurs in children and results from necrotic degeneration of a retropharyngeal lymph node. In adults they can rarely result from the spread of spinal tuberculosis (22). Patients present with stridor, neck stiffness, pain and dysphagia. Protrusion of the posterior pharyngeal wall can be seen on nasendoscopic examination. A full blood count with inflammatory markers and a lateral soft tissue neck radiograph will help confirm the diagnosis, but a CT scan of the neck with contrast is required.

In some situations, a tracheostomy is first performed under local anaesthesia in order to secure the airway, before the abscess is drained via a peroral route.

FOREIGN BODIES (UPPER AERODIGESTIVE TRACT)

Oral cavity – Foreign bodies are usually easily visible on examination with a headlight. It is also possible to palpate the floor of the mouth, tongue and other structures to identify a foreign body. The foreign body can be carefully removed perorally with conventional instruments.

Oropharynx – Foreign bodies, typically fish bones, may not be readily visible. Careful examination of the tonsils, posterior pharyngeal wall, tongue base and valleculae is essential, using both the headlight and flexible nasoendoscope. Visual examination is typically sufficient to exclude a foreign body. However, a lateral soft tissue x-ray is indicated, although some fish bones are not radio-opaque (23). Foreign bodies can be carefully removed per-orally using Magill forceps.

Hypopharynx/oesophagus – Foreign bodies ranging from meat or fish bones, soft food bolus, to batteries and coins can obstruct in this region. Patients will complain of a foreign body sensation, pain, dysphagia or drooling. If the foreign body is above the cricopharyngeus, patients can reliably locate the site of impaction (24).

The most common sites of oesophageal obstruction are at the:

- Cricopharyngeus
- Arch of aorta
- Tracheal bifurcation
- Gastrooesophageal junction.

The hypopharynx can be examined with the flexible nasoendoscope looking carefully in the pyrifom fossae and post-cricoid region. Pooling of saliva in the hypopharynx is suggestive of an oesophageal foreign body.

If the foreign body is not easily visualized in the hypopharynx or oesophagus a soft tissue neck film or chest film (anterior posterior (AP) and lateral) is required. Where a fish bone is difficult to locate CT is more accurate (25, 26).

If the bolus contains no bony or sharp material, these can be initially managed with fizzy drinks or pineapple juice. Buscopan or diazepam can relieve any spasm and allow the bolus to pass into the stomach. If a soft bolus is in the lower oesophagus, then a flexible oesophagogastroduodenoscopy (OGD) is a safer option to push the bolus into the stomach.

If the foreign body is a bone, sharp fragment or non-organic, especially a battery, then removal is required urgently to avoid oesophageal perforation and subsequent complications, including parapharyngeal or mediastinal abscess, which can be fatal.

Larynx/Trachea – A foreign body in the larynx or trachea can cause stridor, voice change, choking, cyanosis, difficulty in breathing, tachypnoea and pneumonia. In an emergency where total or partial obstruction causes compromise, a back slap or abdominal thrust (Heimlich manoeuvre) is employed (27).

In stable patients suspected of having inhaled a foreign body, further investigation is mandatory. In young children, the distinction between ingestion and inhalation is often blurred and they should undergo both chest PA inspiration and expiration views and abdominal films. A senior opinion sought regarding the need for formal endoscopy, which is highly likely.

Most inhaled foreign bodies enter the trachea and then lodge in the right main bronchus.

Foreign bodies at the laryngeal inlet can be removed using an anaesthetic laryngoscope and Magill forceps. Foreign bodies in the trachea and main bronchus require formal tracheobronchoscopy.

LEAKAGE OR LOSS OF TRACHEOESOPHAGEAL VOICE PROSTHESIS

The speech and language therapist or ENT specialist nurse usually undertakes the routine management of the voice prosthesis in patients who have undergone laryngectomy. It is important, however, that all ENT doctors are able to manage a leaking voice prosthesis or inadvertent dislodgement.

In all cases of leakage the patient should be advised to remain nil by mouth until after appropriate assessment to minimize aspiration. To assess the leakage ask the patient to swallow a small sip of coloured fluid (e.g. coloured cordial or food dye in water) while carefully looking at the valve and stoma with a headlight.

Central leakage through the voice prosthesis is the most common. This signifies damage to the valve by *Candida* colonization or inadvertent damage during cleaning of the voice prosthesis. The problem is resolved by fitting a new voice prosthesis by an appropriately trained healthcare professional. If no one is available, the patient is kept nil by mouth and a fine bore feeding tube can be passed through the lumen of the voice prosthesis or a nasogastric tube placed for feeding until a new voice prosthesis can be fitted. If this becomes a recurrent problem, then consideration can be given to fitting a more expensive, anti-fungal voice prosthesis (28, 29).

Peripheral leakage around the voice prosthesis is less common and potentially more difficult to resolve. Leakage is caused by the tracheoesophageal puncture (TEP) becoming larger than the voice prosthesis. This can be related to tumour recurrence or infection, which must be excluded. A number of techniques are available to the appropriately trained individual, including fitting of a larger voice prosthesis, allowing the TEP to shrink and using a smaller voice prosthesis or even removing the voice prosthesis and allowing the TEP to close. If no one suitable is available, the patient is kept nil by mouth and a fine bore feeding tube can be passed through the lumen of the voice prosthesis or a nasogastric tube placed for feeding until such patient can be appropriately managed.

If patients inadvertently dislodge the voice prosthesis, most are taught to pass a dilator, 14Fr Jacques or Foley catheter to keep the TEP patent, or to attend hospital for the same. If the voice prosthesis is not located, then it is prudent to pass a nasoendoscope via the stoma to ensure that the voice prosthesis has not been inhaled. A new voice prosthesis can be fitted by an appropriately trained healthcare professional.

REFERENCES

1 McCarter DF, Courtney AU, Pollart SM. 2007. Cerumen impaction. *Am Fam Physician* 75:1523–8.

2 Burton MJ, Doree C. 2009. Ear drops for the removal of ear wax. *Cochrane Database System Rev* 1: CD004326.

3 SIGN. Diagnosis and management of childhood otitis media in primary care. Available at: www.sign.ac.uk/guidelines/fulltext/66/index. html.

4 NICE. Surgical management of children with otitis media with effusion (OME). Available at: guidance.nice.org.uk/CG60.

5 Geva A, Oestreicher-Kedem Y, Fishman G, Landsberg R, DeRowe A. 2008. Conservative management of acute mastoiditis in children. *Int J Pediatr Otorhinolaryngol* 72: 629–34.

6 Jones SEM, Mahendran S. 2004. Interventions for acute auricular haematoma. *Cochrane Database System Rev* 2: CD004166.

7 Davidi E, Paz A, Duchman H, Luntz M, Potasman I. 2011. Perichondritis of the auricle: Analysis of 114 cases. *Isr Med Assoc J* 13: 21–4.

8 O'Malley MR, Haynes DS. 2008. Sudden hearing loss. *Otolaryngol Clin N Am* 41: 633–49.

9 Wei BPC, Mubiru S, O'Leary S. 2006. Steroids for idiopathic sudden sensorineural hearing loss. *Cochrane Database System Rev* 1: CD003998. doi: 10.1002/14651858. CD003998. pub2.

10 Agarwal L, Pothier DD. 2009. Vasodilators and vasoactive substances for idiopathic sudden sensorineural hearing loss. *Cochrane Database System Rev* 4: CD003422. doi: 10.1002/14651858.CD003422.pub4.

11 Bennett MH, Kertesz T, Perleth M, Yeung P. 2007. Hyperbaric oxygen for idiopathic sudden sensorineural hearing loss and tinnitus. *Cochrane Database System Rev* 1: CD004739. doi: 10.1002/14651858.CD004739. pub3.

12 Danner CJ (2008). Facial nerve paralysis. *Otolaryngol Clin N Am* 41: 619–32.

13 Sullivan FM, Swan IR, Donnan PT et al. 2009. A randomised controlled trial of the use of aciclovir and/or prednisolone for the early treatment of Bell's palsy: The BELLS study. *Health Technol Assess* 13(47): iii–iv, ix–xi, 1–130.

14 Uscategui T, Doree C, Chamberlain IJ, Burton MJ. 2008. Antiviral therapy for Ramsay Hunt syndrome (herpes zoster oticus with facial palsy) in adults. *Cochrane Database System Rev* 4: CD006851. doi: 10.1002/14651858. CD006851.pub2.

15 Uscategui T, Doree C, Chamberlain IJ, Burton MJ. 2008. Corticosteroids as adjuvant to antiviral treatment in Ramsay Hunt syndrome (herpes zoster oticus with facial palsy) in adults. *Cochrane Database System Rev* 3: CD006852. doi: 10.1002/14651858. CD006852. pub2.

16 Little SC, Kesser BW. 2006. Radiographic classification of temporal bone fractures: Clinical predictability using a new system. *Arch Otolaryngol Head Neck Surg* 132: 1300–4.

17 Purohit N, Ray S, Wilson T, Chawla OP. 2008. The 'parent's kiss': An effective way to remove paediatric nasal foreign bodies. *Ann R Coll Surg Engl* 90: 420–22.

18 Chadha NK, Repanos C, Carswell AJ. 2009. Local anaesthesia for manipulation of nasal fractures: Systematic review. *J Laryngol Otol* 123: 830–6.

19 Ketcham AS, Han JK. 2010. Complications and management of septoplasty. *Otolaryngol Clin North Am* 43: 897–904.

20 Guardiani E, Bliss M, Harley E. 2010. Supraglottitis in the era following widespread immunisation against Haemophilus influenzae type B: Evolving principle in diagnosis and management. *Laryngoscope* 120: 2183–8.

21 Sobol SE, Zapata S. 2008. Epiglottitis and Croup. *Otolaryngol Clin N Am* 41: 551–66.

22 Vieira F, Allen SM, Stocks RM, Thompson JW. 2008. Deep neck infection. *Otolaryngol Clin N Am* 41: 459–83.

23 Ell SR, Parker AJ. 1992. The radio-opacity of fishbones. *Clin Otolaryngol Allied Sci* 17(6): 514–6.

24 Connolly AAP, Birchall M, Walsh-Waring GP, Moore-Gillon V. 1992. Ingested foreign bodies: Patient-guided localization is a useful clinical tool. *Clin Otolaryngol Allied Sci* 17(6): 520–4.

25 Lue AJ, Fang WD, Manolidis S. 2000. Use of plain radiography and computed tomography to identify fish bone foreign bodies. *Otolaryngol Head Neck Surg* 123(4): 435–8.

26 Shrime MG, Johnson PE, Stewart MG. 2007. Cost-effective diagnosis of ingested foreign bodies. *Laryngoscope* 117(5): 785–93.

27 UK Resuscitation Council. 2010. Adult basic life support. Resuscitation Guidelines 25–6.

28 Leder SB, Acton LM, Kmiecik J et al. 2005. Voice restoration with the advantage tracheoesophageal voice prosthesis. *Otolaryngol Head Neck Surg* 133(5): 681–4.

29 Soolsma J, van den Brekel MW, Ackerstaff AH et al. 2008. Long-term results of Provox ActiValve, solving the problem of frequent candida- and 'underpressure'- related voice prosthesis replacements. *Laryngoscope* 118(2): 252–7.

4 EPISTAXIS

Joanne Rimmer

INTRODUCTION

This common ENT emergency has been estimated to affect 7%–14% of the population at some point, but ENT specialists see only around 6% of all cases (1). Patients may present in the acute setting, or may be seen on an elective basis in the outpatient clinic with recurrent episodes of epistaxis.

ANATOMY

Multiple branches of both the internal and external carotid arteries supply the nose, through multiple anastamoses. The internal carotid artery supplies the superior nasal cavity via the anterior and posterior ethmoid arteries which are branches of the ophthalmic artery. The external carotid supplies the nasal cavity via the superior labial, lateral nasal and ascending palatine branches of the facial artery and the sphenopalatine, ascending pharyngeal and greater palatine branches of the maxillary artery (2).

Most epistaxis arises from the septum rather than the lateral wall of the nose. The most common site of bleeding is Little's area on the anterior septum, also known as Kiesselbach's plexus (Figure 4.1) (3).

Woodruff's plexus (a venous plexus located inferior to the posterior end of the inferior turbinate) has been described as a common site of posterior bleeding (4), but it is now accepted that even posterior bleeds are more likely to be septal than from the lateral nasal wall (5).

AETIOLOGY

Epistaxis can be classified into primary (idiopathic), or secondary to a specific cause such as trauma (6). Around 80% of epistaxis is idiopathic. Causative factors can be divided into local and systemic (Table 4.1).

The most commonly identified local cause of epistaxis is trauma – digital, surgical or accidental. Other local causes include infection, inflammation, foreign body, endocrine (e.g. pregnancy), benign

(e.g. juvenile nasopharyngeal angiofibroma) or malignant sinonasal tumours or environmental (e.g. airborne particulate matter) (7).

Systemic causes include antiplatelet or anticoagulant drugs (e.g. aspirin, clopidogrel, warfarin, heparin), haematological disorders (e.g. haemophilia, leukaemia, thrombocytopenia), liver failure and hereditary haemorrhagic telangiectasia (HHT).

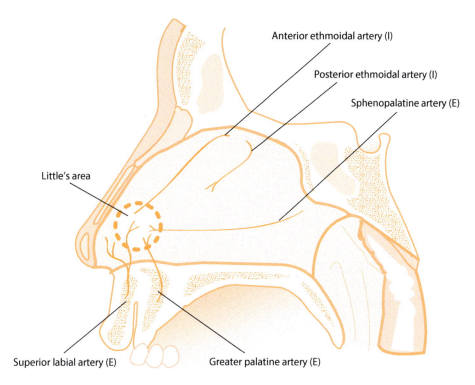

Anterior ethmoidal artery (I)

Posterior ethmoidal artery (I)

Sphenopalatine artery (E)

Little's area

Superior labial artery (E)

Greater palatine artery (E)

Figure 4.1. Arterial blood supply to the nose. The nose has a rich blood supply, by both internal (I) and external (E) carotid arteries. Little's area, or Kiesselbach's plexus, represents a confluence of these vessels.

Table 4.1. Local and systemic causes of epistaxis.

Local	Systemic
Trauma	Drugs (e.g. aspirin, clopidogrel, warfarin)
Infection (e.g. URTI, acute rhinosinusitis)	Haematological disorders (e.g. haemophilia, leukaemia, thrombocytopaenia)
Inflammation (e.g. rhinitis)	
Foreign body	Liver failure
Endocrine (e.g. pregnancy)	Hereditary haemorrhagic telangiectasia (HHT)
Neoplastic (benign or malignant)	

HISTORY

In the elective outpatient setting this can be taken at leisure; in an acute bleed it is often done whilst treatment is being initiated. Important points about the bleeding itself include onset, duration, side (may often start on one side then appear to become bilateral due to overflow), whether anterior (running out of the nose) or posterior (swallowing blood) – although it may be both with profuse bleeding, previous episodes and any treatment given and precipitating factors, including recent trauma or surgery. If trauma is involved, significant head injury must be excluded.

Key factors in the past medical history include hypertension, coagulopathies and HHT. Relevant drugs include antihypertensives, antiplatelet agents and anticoagulants. Social history is important as it may determine whether a patient is safe to be discharged after a significant bleed – a frail elderly patient living alone may not be.

MANAGEMENT

Never underestimate this ENT emergency as it can be life-threatening. Always begin with the ABC algorithm:

Airway – Examine the oropharynx and suction any clots
Breathing
Circulation – Ensure wide-bore intravenous access and send blood for a full blood count and group and save in all but minor cases; routine coagulation screens are not indicated in the absence of relevant risk factors (8). Check heart rate and blood pressure and resuscitate with fluids and/or blood as required. Remember young patients may maintain a normal pulse rate and blood pressure until in severe shock. Estimate blood loss and instigate simple first aid measures with firm compression of both nostrils, head tilted forward, and apply ice to the back of the patient's neck.

EXAMINATION

In the outpatient clinic (or if the acute bleed has settled) this can be done thoroughly. In the acute situation it may not be possible to fully examine the patient, depending on the degree of bleeding.

If you are able to do so, begin with anterior rhinoscopy using a Thudichum's speculum and headlight. This allows inspection of the anterior septum including Little's area, a likely site of the bleeding vessel. If no obvious bleeding point is seen and the situation permits, complete the examination using a rigid 0° Hopkins rod endoscope to evaluate both nasal cavities and postnasal space.

In emergency situations, wear gloves, an eye shield, and an apron or gown. Suction is required during examination and treatment, and other equipment should be available to allow further management, as detailed below.

TREATMENT

It is important to correct over-anticoagulation and hypertension, and medical or haematological input may be required. Thrombocytopaenia should be corrected with platelet transfusion; packs should be avoided if possible as they cause further trauma to the nasal mucosa with inevitable rebleeding on removal. Absorbable packs, such as oxidized cellulose or gelatin sponge soaked in adrenaline or tranexamic acid, are a useful alternative. There is little to be gained from stopping aspirin therapy as the half-life of platelets is seven days, but if a warfarinized patient has a significantly elevated INR then withholding warfarin is advisable until the bleeding is controlled and the INR back in the therapeutic range. The use of low dose diazepam has been advocated in the past, particularly in anxious hypertensive patients, but there is little evidence for its use; controlling the epistaxis is more effective in reducing both blood pressure and anxiety (9).

See Figure 4.2 for a basic treatment algorithm for epistaxis.

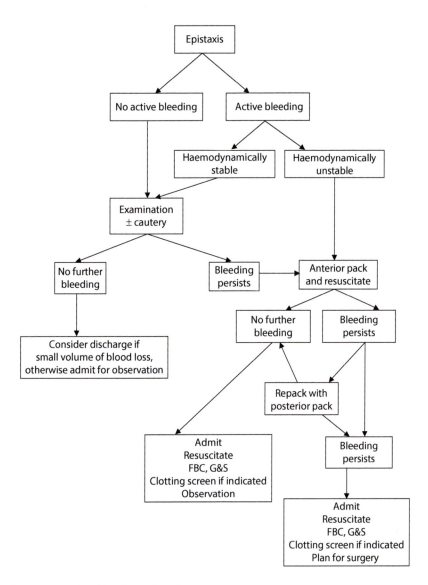

Figure 4.2. A treatment algorithm for epistaxis.

CAUTERY

The ideal management option is to identify and cauterize the bleeding vessel. This controls the epistaxis, avoids packing and in many cases allows the patient to be discharged. As most bleeding vessels arise in Little's area, silver nitrate cautery is often possible with anterior rhinoscopy.

The bleeding vessel is identified and topical anaesthesia, ideally combined with a vasoconstrictor (e.g. co-phenylcaine – 5% lidocaine with 0.5% phenylephrine), is applied on cotton wool. Silver nitrate cautery of the vessel is then performed directly; if it is an 'end-on' vessel, it can be helpful to cauterize around it before touching the vessel itself. Naseptin™ cream (0.1% chlorhexidine dihydrochloride, 0.5% neomycin sulphate) is applied to the cauterized area twice daily for two weeks. An alternative, such as chloramphenicol ointment, should be used in patients with peanut allergy, as Naseptin™ contains arachis (peanut) oil.

If an obvious vessel or bleeding point is not seen anteriorly, it may be possible to examine more posteriorly with a rigid endoscope. Whilst the use of silver nitrate cautery is possible for posterior epistaxis, it is more difficult to be precise and avoid touching other parts of the nose with the stick (10). If available, bipolar electrocautery is more practical for use with an endoscope, allowing diathermy of the specific bleeding point (11).

ANTERIOR NASAL PACKING

If the epistaxis is not controlled with simple measures, then packing is required. In the first instance this is anterior nasal packing, which is most commonly performed with a nasal tampon. Various anterior packs are available, from simple sponges such as Merocel™ to newer self-lubricating hydrocolloid-covered packs such as Rapid Rhino™.

The insertion technique is the same for all types. The nasal tip is elevated with one hand and the pack pushed firmly in along the floor of the nose with the other. It is preferable to support the back of the patient's head to facilitate complete insertion in one smooth movement. Ensure that the pack is inserted parallel to the palate as the nasal cavity runs straight back, not upwards (Figure 4.3(a)). Once in place, sponges need to

be inflated with a little water; newer devices have a concealed balloon that requires inflation (Figure 4.3(b)).

Unilateral packing of the bleeding side may be sufficient. However, the expanded pack may simply push the septum across without providing adequate compression. If bleeding continues, a contralateral pack should be inserted.

Anterior packing may also be performed with a long length of ribbon gauze soaked in bismuth iodoform paraffin paste (BIPP). This is layered into the nose, along its whole length, using Tilley dressing forceps (Figure 4.4). This is not a pleasant experience for the patient whose head will need supporting posteriorly during the packing, but it can be a very effective

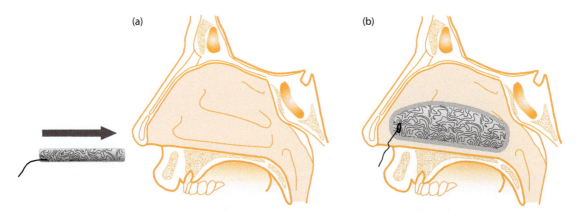

Figure 4.3. (a) Insertion of a nasal pack. (b) A nasal pack in situ.

Figure 4.4. BIPP ribbon gauze packing of the nasal cavity.

way of providing more compression than nasal tampons.

It is standard practice in most departments to admit patients once they have been packed, for observation and pack removal within 24 hours, if stable. However, local protocols will be in place, and some patients may be discharged with their pack(s) in situ, to return for follow-up and pack removal in the outpatient department (12).

Recent studies have reported the use of a haemostatic matrix to control epistaxis, as a successful alternative to anterior nasal packing (13). These commercially available products contain gelatin $\pm$ human thrombin and are prepared in a syringe, which allows easy instillation into the nose. If bleeding is controlled, patients do not require hospital admission.

POSTERIOR NASAL PACKING

If bleeding continues despite adequate anterior nasal packing, the next step is a posterior pack. There are various commercial balloon devices designed for this (Figure 4.5). Although not licensed for this use, a female Foley catheter (size 12 or 14 French) is an alternative. The catheter is passed along the floor of the nose until the tip is seen behind the soft palate. Once inflated with 5–10 mL of water (not saline as this can corrode the balloon), the catheter is gently pulled back into

Figure 4.5. Inflated epistaxis balloon in situ.

the posterior choana. The catheter is clipped to prevent deflation of the balloon and to hold it in place; an umbilical clip or a simple artery clip can be used. An anterior BIPP pack is placed around the catheter. It is essential to ensure that the catheter or clip does not rest on the nares as they can rapidly cause pressure necrosis of the alar rim with subsequent notching. Gauze or cotton wool should be used to protect the alar margin.

Other complications reported with posterior nasal packing are respiratory (e.g. obstructive sleep apnoea), vagal (from nasopharyngeal stimulation) and cardiac (including myocardial infarction) (14). Patients who require posterior packing need close observation as it implies significant epistaxis.

Packs, either anterior or posterior are left in for up to 24 hours and no longer than 48 hours. If the patient has any risk factors for endocarditis, oral antibiotic cover (e.g. amoxicillin) is given while packs are in place.

SURGICAL INTERVENTION

If bleeding remains uncontrolled, or if the patient bleeds again after removal of their pack, an examination under anaesthetic is required with a view to cautery or vessel ligation, as indicated, or rarely more formal posterior nasal packing.

Septoplasty may be required if there is significant deviation or a large septal spur; this may have prevented adequate packing initially. If an obvious bleeding point is seen it can be cauterized with bipolar diathermy.

VESSEL LIGATION

Endoscopic sphenopalatine artery (SPA) ligation is now commonly employed as the primary surgical procedure for epistaxis when operative intervention is required (15). The SPA is the major blood supply to the posterior aspect of the nasal cavity, and may have multiple branches that require ligating individually.

Transantral maxillary artery ligation, via a Caldwell Luc approach in most cases, has become less popular with the advent of the endoscopic SPA technique, which is much less invasive.

If SPA/maxillary artery ligation fails to control bleeding, or in cases of traumatic epistaxis (with possible ethmoid fracture), then the anterior and posterior ethmoid arteries can be ligated. This is performed via an external approach using a modified Lynch–Howarth incision.

If bleeding continues despite these measures, then the external carotid artery may be ligated in the neck (16).

EMBOLIZATION

Some centres will have access to radiological embolization. This may be employed if other measures have failed, or if general anaesthesia must be avoided due to significant comorbidities. Patients must be actively bleeding for this procedure, as angiography is required to identify the bleeding vessel before particulate embolization can be performed. Patients must be warned of the risk of stroke, skin and palate necrosis (17).

HEREDITARY HAEMORRHAGIC TELANGIECTASIA

This autosomal dominant condition warrants specific mention, as its most common symptom is epistaxis. There are multiple telangiectasias of the nasal mucosa which are very fragile and bleed with minimal trauma. Patients are generally well-informed and will often not seek medical treatment unless the bleeding becomes severe or protracted. Cautery and nasal packing should be avoided if at all possible. If packing is required, an absorbable pack such as a gelatin sponge soaked in adrenaline is the most appropriate method, as the nasal mucosa will be further traumatized by pack insertion and subsequent removal. If formal packing is required, it should ideally be removed in theatre under general anaesthetic, when potassium titanyl phosphate (KTP) or argon laser can be used to target the individual lesions, or more definitive treatment such as septodermoplasty or nasal closure can be performed (18). Vessel ligation and embolization provide only a temporary solution, but may allow time to arrange for more definitive treatment as above. Such cases may require discussion with a specialist centre.

KEY POINTS:

- Epistaxis is a common problem that is potentially life-threatening; resuscitation may be required.
- Cautery of the bleeding point is often successful, as most primary epistaxis arises from the anterior septum.
- Anterior with or without posterior nasal packing may be required to control profuse bleeding.
- Recalcitrant cases require timely operative intervention.

REFERENCES

1 McGarry GW. 2008. Epistaxis. In: Gleeson MJ, editor. *Scott-Brown's Otorhinolaryngology Head & Neck Surgery*. 7th ed. Hodder Arnold, London.

2 Janfaza P, Montgomery WW, Salman SD. 2001. Nasal cavities and paranasal sinuses. In: Janfaza P, Nadol JB, Galla RJ, Fabian RL, Montgomery WW, editors. *Surgical Anatomy of the Head and Neck*. Lippincott Williams & Wilkins, Philadelphia.

3 Mackenzie D. 1914. Little's area or the Locus Kiesselbachi. *J Laryngol* 1: 21–2.

4 Woodruff GH. 1949. Cardiovascular epistaxis and the naso-nasopharyngeal plexus. *Laryngoscope* 15: 1238–47.

5 Chiu TW, Shaw-Dunn J, McGarry GW. 1998. Woodruff's naso-nasopharyngeal plexus: How important is it in posterior epistaxis? *Clin Otolaryngol* 23: 272–9.

6 Melia L, McGarry GW. 2011. Epistaxis: Update on management. *Curr Op Otolaryngol Head Neck Surg* 19: 30–5.

7 Bray D, Monnery P, Toma AG. 2004. Airborne environmental pollutant concentration and hospital epistaxis presentation: A 5-year review. *Clin Otolaryngol* 29: 655–8.

8 Shakeel M, Trinidade A, Iddamalgoda T, Supriya M, Ah-See KW. 2010. Routine clotting screen has no role in the management of epistaxis: Reiterating the point. *Eur Archiv Otorhinolaryngol* 267: 1641–4.

9 Thong JF, Lo S, Houghton R, Moore-Gillon V. 2007. A prospective comparative study to examine the effects of oral diazepam on blood pressure and anxiety levels in patients with acute epistaxis. *J Laryngol Otol* 121: 124–9.

10 Webb CJ, Beer H. 2004. Posterior nasal cautery with silver nitrate. *J Laryngol Otol* 118: 713–4.

11 Ahmed A, Woolford TJ. 2003. Endoscopic bipolar diathermy in the management of epistaxis: An effective and cost-efficient treatment. *Clin Otolaryngol* 28: 273–5.

12 Van Wyk FC, Massey S, Worley G, Brady S. 2007. Do all epistaxis patients with a nasal pack need admission? A retrospective study of 116 patients managed in accident and emergency with a peer-reviewed protocol. *J Laryngol Otol* 121: 222–7.

13 Mathiasen RA, Cruz RM. 2005. Prospective, randomized, controlled clinical trial of a novel matrix hemostatic sealant in patients with acute anterior epistaxis. *Laryngoscope* 115: 899–902.

14 Rotenberg B, Tam S. 2010. Respiratory complications from nasal packing: Systematic review. *J Otolaryngol Head Neck Surg* 39: 606–14.

15 Douglas R, Wormald P. 2007. Update on epistaxis. *Curr Op Otolaryngol Head Neck Surg* 15: 180–3.

16 Srinivasan V, Sherman IW, O'Sullivan G. 2000. Surgical management of intractable epistaxis: An audit of results. *J Laryngol Otol* 114: 697–700.

17 Sadri M, Midwinter K, Ahmed A, Parker A. 2006. Assessment of safety and efficacy of arterial embolization in the management of intractable epistaxis. *Eur Archiv Otorhinolaryngol* 263: 560–6.

18 Rimmer J, Lund VJ. 2015. Hereditary haemorrhagic telangiectasia. *Rhinology* 53: 195–203.

5
AUDIOLOGY

Neil Donnelly

The principal function of audiological testing is to establish hearing thresholds accurately and to determine whether there is any impairment. If impairment is detected, testing is used to establish the site, type (conductive, sensorineural or mixed) and severity of the hearing loss (Figure 5.1).

Tests of hearing are divided into behavioural and objective. When presented with sound, each aspect of the auditory pathway responds in a way that can be measured. This response may be the test subject performing a specific task to indicate hearing a sound stimulus (behavioural response) or the measurement of a physical property of the

Figure 5.1. Levels of hearing loss.

system (objective response). Objective tests do not require the active cooperation of a subject and are not a true measure of hearing, which is a subjective sensation. They do, however, allow for certain inferences to be made regarding a subject's ability to hear.

BEHAVIOURAL AUDIOMETRY

▋ Pure tone audiometry

Indication

● To establish hearing thresholds.

Pure tone audiometry is used to provide threshold information and to identify the presence and magnitude of any hearing loss. Thresholds are usually measured both for air conduction (via headphones) and for bone conduction (via a bone vibrator). The information provided by pure tone audiometry may be plotted graphically as an audiogram. The audiogram represents hearing sensitivity (dB HL) across a discrete frequency spectrum (125–8000 Hz). A wide variety of symbols are used to denote the findings (Figure 5.2).

O	Right air conduction thresholds
X	Left air conduction thresholds
Δ	Unmasked bone conduction
[	Right bone conduction thresholds
]	Left bone conduction thresholds
↘	Threshold poorer at that level, but cannot be determined because of limited output of the audiometer

Figure 5.2. Symbols commonly used in pure tone audiometry.

The reason for using a hearing level scale rather than sound pressure level (SPL) scale reflects the fact that the threshold of hearing as measured in SPL is not the same across all frequencies. For example, less energy is required to detect a 1000 Hz sound at threshold (7.5 dB SPL) than at 125 Hz (47.5 dB SPL); the resulting audiogram would be particularly difficult to interpret. The dB HL scale

is a scale of human hearing where 0 dB HL reflects the threshold of hearing of an otologically normal individual irrespective of its frequency. It is against this normal hearing population that an individual's hearing is compared.

Pure tone audiometry is performed in accordance with the British Society of Audiology's recommended procedures (1). Testing is ideally carried out in a sound proof acoustic booth to minimize background noise. Frequency-specific sound stimuli are first delivered via headphones to test air conduction thresholds. Patients are instructed to indicate (by pressing a button) when they hear a tone, however faint. Testing begins with the better hearing ear and frequencies (250–8000 Hz) are tested in a specified order. Stimuli are initially presented at 30 dB above expected threshold. This is increased in 20 dB steps if not initially heard. The stimulus is then lowered in 10 dB steps until no longer heard and raised in 5 dB steps until a threshold becomes evident. There must be a minimum of two responses at that level. The threshold is marked on the audiogram with the appropriate symbol. Bone conduction thresholds are undertaken with a bone vibrator placed on the mastoid process of the ear with the worst air conduction thresholds. It is only possible to test frequencies between 250 and 4000 Hz. The maximum output of the bone vibrator is approximately 70 dB; stimulation beyond these levels may result in the vibrations being felt rather than heard.

Air conduction thresholds represent the sensitivity of the hearing mechanism as a whole (conductive, sensorineural and central components), whereas bone conduction thresholds represent the sensitivity of the hearing mechanism from the cochlear onwards. Any difference between the two thresholds is referred to as an air–bone gap

(ABG). An ABG is attributed to a problem in the conduction mechanism and hence referred to as a conductive hearing loss.

In reality, sound through bone conduction reaches the cochlea in three ways:

1 Sound escapes to the external ear canal and is subsequently transferred to the cochlea through the normal middle ear mechanism.
2 Vibrations travel directly through the middle ear ossicles and then to the cochlea.
3 Vibrations reach the cochlea directly through the skull.

If there is an external or middle ear pathology resulting in a conductive hearing loss, sound will be poorly transmitted by the first two routes, resulting in poorer bone conduction thresholds than expected. This effect is greatest at 2 kHz and explains the Carhart notch seen in otosclerosis. It also explains why correcting a conductive hearing loss can result in an apparent over closure in the bone conduction thresholds.

As discussed above, pure tone audiometry presents sound to one ear at a time, and the response measured. However, in certain conditions it is not possible to be certain that the intended (test) ear is the one actually responding. In some cases the non-test ear can pick up the sound just as well or better, a phenomenon known as cross-hearing (Figure 5.3).

For example, when the hearing acuity of the ears is very different it is possible that when testing the worse ear, the better ear detects the test signal more easily. In this situation special techniques (masking) are employed to 'exclude' the non-test ear.

In order to understand cross-hearing it is necessary to understand how sound travels to the cochlea during audiological testing using the headphones and the bone vibrator. When a sound is presented via headphones to one ear, part of the energy escapes and vibrates the skull. This sound energy is transmitted via bone conduction to the cochlea of the opposite side and is attenuated (loses sound energy) by approximately 40 dB (Figure 5.3(a)).

A bone vibrator, on the other hand will vibrate the entire skull regardless of where it is placed, with sound energy being transmitted to both cochleas with little or no attenuation (0 dB). It therefore corresponds to the best hearing cochlea, regardless of the side tested (Figure 5.3(b)). For this reason, it is the sensitivity of the better hearing cochlea that determines whether masking is required, not the better hearing ear.

The three particular rules are employed to help determine whether masking is needed (2).

▌ Rules of masking

Rule 1 – When testing air conduction, if the threshold between the two ears differs by 40 dB or more at any frequency, the worse ear becomes the test ear and the better ear is masked.
Rule 2 – When testing bone conduction, if the not-masked bone conduction threshold at any frequency is better than the worse ear air conduction threshold by 10 dB or more, the worse ear by air conduction becomes the test ear and the better ear is masked. This provides ear-specific masked bone conduction thresholds.
Rule 3 – When testing air conduction, if rule 1 has not been applied (i.e. interaural AC

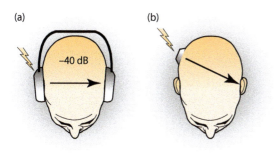

(a) (b)

−40 dB

Figure 5.3. (a) Transcranial attenuation through air and (b) bone conduction.

difference less than 40 dB), but the not-masked bone conduction threshold is better by 40 dB, then the not-masked air conduction is attributed to the worse ear. The worse ear becomes the test ear and the better ear is then masked.

Interpretation of an audiogram

- Air and bone conduction thresholds equal to or better than 20 dB are considered to be within normal limits (Figure 5.4(a)). Beyond 20 dB, the degree of hearing loss is classified as mild, moderate, severe or profound (Figure 5.4(a–d)).
- With a pure conductive hearing loss, the ear specific masked bone conduction threshold is normal while there is a gap of more than 10 dB between the air and bone conduction thresholds (Figure 5.4(b)). This gap is known as the air–bone gap (ABG).
- With a pure sensorineural hearing loss, both the ear-specific air and the bone conduction thresholds are worse than 20 dB, but there is no ABG (Figure 5.4(c)).

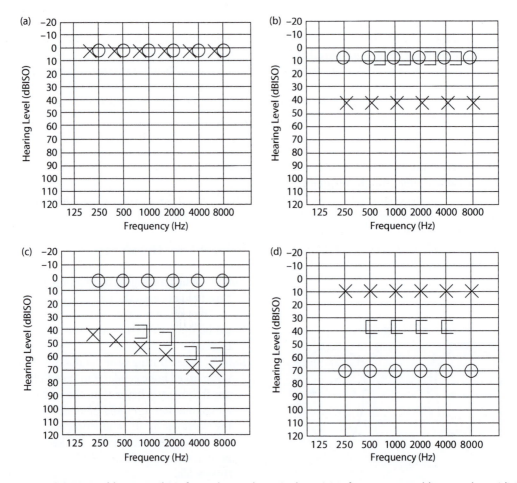

Figure 5.4. (a) Normal hearing. (b) Left conductive hearing loss. (c) Left sensorineural hearing loss. (d) Right mixed hearing loss.

- In a mixed hearing loss, the ear-specific bone conduction thresholds are worse than 20 dB and there is an ABG greater than 10 dB (Figure 5.4(d)).

- Asymmetry in thresholds is considered significant if there is more than 10 dB difference between the ears at two adjacent frequencies.

SPEECH AUDIOMETRY

Indications

- Functional hearing assessment (speech or word discrimination).
- To confirm conductive or sensorineural hearing loss.
- Investigation of non-organic hearing loss.

In speech audiometry, the patient is asked to repeat pre-recorded words (i.e. the Arthur Boothroyd word list) presented via a free field, headphones or bone conductor at various intensity levels. The speech audiogram graphically displays the percentage of correct responses as a function of the sound pressure level that the words were presented at (Figure 5.5). One of the variables measured is the optimum discrimination score (ODS). This is 100% in patients with normal hearing (line 1, Figure 5.5) and in patients with pure conductive hearing losses, although a conductive loss requires higher intensity levels

(line 2, Figure 5.5). In sensorineural hearing losses, ODS is usually less than 100%, regardless of the sound intensity (line 3, Figure 5.5). With neural losses, a phenomenon known as roll-over may be observed (line 4, Figure 5.5).

Speech audiometry supplies useful information regarding a patient's hearing handicap and can guide management of the condition. An example of this is in the management of otosclerosis. When considering stapedectomy, a patient with an ODS of less than 70% must be counselled that their perceived benefit may not be as good as that of someone with a score of over 70%, even if the ABG is successfully closed. An optimum discrimination score of less than 50% is regarded as being not socially useful, which can have implications in the management of individuals with vestibular schwannoma. If optimally aided ODS in the better hearing ear is less than 50%, then an individual may meet the criteria for cochlear implantation.

Figure 5.5. Speech audiogram.

▌ Tympanometry

Indications

- In conjunction with audiometry to characterize hearing loss.
- To document normal middle ear compliance.

Tympanometry is not a test of hearing, but is used in conjunction with pure tone audiometry to help determine the nature of any hearing loss.

Tympanometry measures the compliance of the middle ear system. Factors influencing middle ear compliance include the integrity and mobility of the tympanic membrane and ossicular chain, the presence of fluid and middle ear pressure. Tympanometry is therefore used clinically to provide information regarding the state of the tympanic membrane, ossicular chain, middle ear cleft and Eustachian tube function.

The test involves placing a small probe in the ear canal to form an airtight seal. The probe contains a sound generator, microphone and pump, all connected to a tympanometer. A sound stimulus is passed down the ear canal to the tympanic membrane. The stimulus used is a 226 Hz probe tone unless testing infants less than four months old, for whom a 1 kHz stimulus is used. A proportion of the sound energy is transmitted through the middle ear apparatus and the rest is reflected. The probe microphone records reflected sound energy. The more compliant the middle ear system, the less energy reflected. Because the compliance of the tympanic membrane is maximal when the pressure between its two sides is equal, it is possible to measure the middle ear pressure by altering the pressure in the external ear canal via the pump channel in the ear probe.

The test generates a tympanogram. This is a graphical representation of the compliance of the tympanic membrane as a function of the change in pressure in the external ear canal. Tympanograms are most commonly described according to the Jerger system of classification (3). There are three types:

Type A – Demonstrates a well-defined peak compliance of between +100 and −150 daPa (Figure 5.6(a)). It signifies normal middle ear pressure.

Type B – Demonstrating no obvious peak across the pressure range (Figure 5.6(b)). Interpretation depends on the measured ear

(a) Type A   (b) Type B   (c) Type C

Figure 5.6. Tympanometry. (a) Normal peak. (b) No peak. (c) Negative peak.

canal volume. This should be less than 1 cm³ in a child and less than 1.5 cm³ in an adult. If the ear canal volume is normal, the flat trace is likely to represent a middle ear effusion. If the ear canal volume is increased, then the finding is likely to represent a tympanic membrane perforation or presence of a patent grommet.

Type C – Demonstrates a well-defined compliance peak at less than −150 daPa (Figure 5.6(c)). This most commonly signifies Eustachian tube dysfunction or a partial middle ear effusion.

Tympanometry does not provide information about hearing, and inferences must be made in conjunction with information from other tests.

AUDITORY EVOKED POTENTIALS

Indications

- To establish likely hearing thresholds.
- To identify cochlear or retro-cochlear pathology.

Auditory evoked potentials (AEPs) describe the electrical activity within the cochlea and along the auditory pathway in response to auditory stimulation. The test involves a sound stimulus being presented to the test ear. This results in electrical activity within the auditory pathway. Scalp electrodes detect this and other non-auditory activity. The electrodes pass information to an amplifier which amplifies and filters differences between pairs of electrodes. The stimulus is presented repeatedly and the recordings averaged. The process of amplification, filtering and averaging results in evoked potential (signal) being separated from non-auditory electrical activity (noise).

Four types of AEP are in common clinical usage:

1 *Electrocochleography* – This measures electrical activity within the cochlea and first-order cochlear nerve fibres in response to sound. The electrocochleogram (ECochG) records three potentials: the cochlear microphonic (CM), the summating potential (SP) and the action potential (AP). Common clinical uses include frequency-specific estimation of hearing thresholds in the very young or difficult to test and the determination of endolymphatic hydrops in Ménière's disease.

2 *Auditory brainstem responses (ABR)* – The auditory brainstem response is a series of five waves occurring within 10 ms of a sound stimulus (Figure 5.7). Each wave is attributed to a different part of the auditory pathway from distal auditory nerve to inferior colliculus.

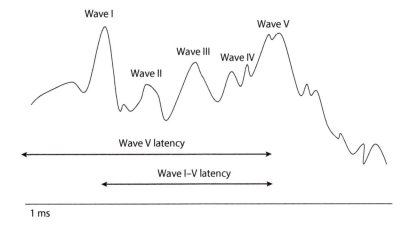

Figure 5.7. Auditory brainstem response in waves.

ABR has a number of clinical uses, principally the estimation of hearing thresholds using wave V. Because the ABR is present from birth it is a useful hearing screening tool for neonates. The precise latency of each waveform has previously been exploited to detect pathology affecting the cochlear nerve, in particular as a screening test for vestibular schwannomas. In this condition there can be a delay in the latency of wave V. This has now been superseded by contrast-enhanced magnetic resonance imaging (MRI).

3 *Auditory steady state responses (ASSR)* – This is a test that uses frequency-specific stimuli modulated with respect to amplitude and frequency. Higher modulation rates generate AEP derived from the brainstem. Auditory steady state responses (ASSR) analysis is based on the fact that related electrical activity coincides with the stimulus repetition rate and relies on statistical detection algorithms. The test can be used as an automated assessment of auditory thresholds.

4 *Cortical auditory evoked potentials (CAEPs)* – Evoked potentials occurring beyond 50 ms are referred to as CAEPs. They span the transition from obligatory to cognitive responses. They can be generated using frequency stimuli. The accurate correspondence with true frequency-specific hearing thresholds make this a useful test in medico-legal assessment of hearing for compensation cases and for diagnosis in suspected non-organic hearing loss.

OTOACOUSTIC EMISSIONS

Indications

● Hearing screening.

Otoacoustic emissions (OAEs) represent sound energy generated by the contraction and expansion of outer hair cells in the cochlear. These echoes can be measured by sensitive microphones placed in the ear canal. OAEs are classified into two groups: spontaneous (only present in 50% of population) and evoked. Evoked OAEs are emissions generated in response to a sound stimulus and are present in the majority of individuals with hearing thresholds better that 40 dB HL. In fact, OAEs are present in 99% of individuals with thresholds better than 20 dB and always absent with thresholds over 40 dB. Between 20 and 40 dB there is a zone of uncertainty. For this reason they have been widely adopted as a hearing screening tool (4).

Clinically, two main types of evoked OAEs are used: transient evoked OAEs (TEOAEs) and distortion product OAEs (DPOAEs). The test involves placing a small insert in the ear canal, which contains a sound generator and microphone and is attached to an OAE machine. A stimulus is generated and any ensuing emission measured. The test is performed in a quiet environment. In addition to being able to infer hearing thresholds of better than 40 dB HL, these tests provide frequency-specific information in the speech frequencies (500–4000 Hz).

Absent evoked OAEs do not necessarily reflect a cochlear hearing loss and can arise if the ear canal is blocked or if there is middle ear pathology (i.e. an effusion). If OAEs are genuinely absent, no inference as to the degree of loss can be made, which can range from mild (zone of uncertainty) to profound. Additionally, robust OAEs may be found in individuals with auditory neuropathy spectrum disorder, who may have a profound hearing loss.

KEY POINTS:

- Ensure testing equipment is maintained and meets the appropriate National Physical Laboratory calibration schedule.
- Expertise is required for both the testing and interpretation of results.
- Ensure that appropriate ear-specific information is obtained. Have masking rules been applied?
- No single test provides all the answers.
- Beware of discrepancies. Where outcomes of tests are unexpected and do not fit with observed auditory function, check that the equipment is functioning normally and that the test subject is performing the test appropriately.

✱ RECOMMENDED READING

- Browning GG (2nd edition 1998). *Clinical Otology & Audiology*. Butterworth-Heinemann, London.

- Graham J, Baguley D. 2009. *Ballantyne's Deafness*. Wiley-Blackwell, Chichester.
- Katz J, Medwetsky L, Buckard RF, Hood LJ 6th edition 2010). *Handbook of Clinical Audiology*. Lippincott Williams & Wilkins.

REFERENCES

1 British Society of Audiology. 1981. Recommended procedures for pure-tone audiometry using a manually operated instrument. *Br J Audiol* 15: 213–6.
2 British Society of Audiology. 1986. Recommendations procedures for masking in pure tone threshold audiometry. *Br J Audiol* 20: 307–14.
3 Jerger J. 1970. Clinical experience with impedance audiometry. *Arch Otolaryngol* 92: 311–24.
4 Rea PA, Gibson WP. 2003. Evidence for surviving outer hair cell function in congenitally deaf ears. *Laryngoscope* 113: 2030–4.

TONSILLECTOMY

James Tysome

Indications

- Recurrent acute tonsillitis.
- Two or more episodes of quinsy.
- Obstructive sleep apnoea.
- Possible malignancy (e.g. unilateral tonsillar enlargement or ulceration of the tonsil surface).
- In cases of an unknown primary (i.e. a metastatic deposit in a neck lymph node), tonsillectomy may be indicated in order to exclude this as a site for the primary in conjunction with a panendoscopy.
- As part of an uvulopalatopharyngoplasty performed for the treatment of snoring.
- To access a parapharyngeal abscess.
- Rarely to access an elongated styloid process in the management of Eagle syndrome.

Recurrent acute tonsillitis remains the commonest indication for tonsillectomy. The frequency and severity of episodes required to list a patient for this procedure varies from unit to unit. Whilst the Scottish Intercollegiate Guidelines Network (SIGN) recommendations are helpful (suggesting patients who suffer five or more episodes of tonsillitis per annum benefit from this procedure) a decision must be made on a case-by-case basis (1, 2).

PREOPERATIVE REVIEW

The vascularity of the tonsillar tissue increases significantly during an episode of tonsillitis. Many surgeons will postpone surgery if the patient has experienced true tonsillitis in the preceding 28 days, even if antibiotics have been prescribed, as intra-operative haemorrhage is increased if tonsillectomy is performed.

OPERATIVE PROCEDURE

Once anaesthetized and the airway secured with an endotracheal tube (ET), a shoulder bolster is placed under the patient and the neck extended. The patient's eyes must be taped closed. A headlight is worn by the surgeon and the patient draped.

The operation is performed from the head of the operating table. A Boyle–Davis mouth gag with an appropriately-sized blade is inserted and the mouth gently opened. The tongue is positioned in the midline by sweeping the tongue base with digital manipulation. Draffin rods are used to support and lift the gag. The head must remain supported on the operating table.

Secretions are cleared from the oral cavity using suction (Figure 6.1(a)).

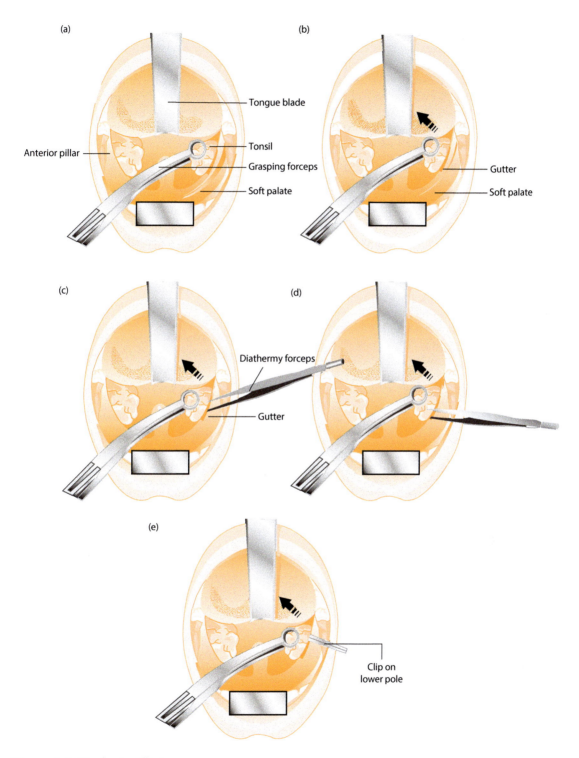

(a)

Tongue blade

Anterior pillar

Tonsil

Grasping forceps

Soft palate

(b)

Gutter

Soft palate

(c)

Diathermy forceps

Gutter

(d)

(e)

Clip on
lower pole

Figure 6.1. Bipolar tonsillectomy.

In order to remove the right tonsil, Dennis–Brown or Luc's forceps are held in the surgeon's left hand and the superior pole of the right tonsil is gently grasped and pulled medially (Figure 6.1(b)). This, in most cases, produces a visible gutter in the anterior tonsillar pillar, which marks the lateral limit of the tonsil. The mucosa is incised using McIndoe scissors or cauterized with bipolar forceps (Figure 6.1(c)). The scissors can then be gently inserted into the incision and opened to develop the plane between the tonsil and the superior constrictor muscle fibres. At this stage, the forceps are repositioned with the superior blade within this developed plane and the inferior blade over the medial surface of the tonsil.

A Gwynne–Evans dissector or bipolar diathermy forceps may be used to separate the muscle fibres from the white capsule of the tonsil, which should gradually peel away. Bleeding is inevitable during this part of the procedure but identifying the tonsillar capsule early and staying within the correct plane will minimize its extent. Continued traction with the forceps is the key to a clean and brisk dissection (Figure 6.1(d)).

As the dissection proceeds, a small 'stalk' of tissue tethers the tonsil at its inferior pole. This usually bears a significant feeding arterial vessel (the tonsillar branch of the ascending pharyngeal artery) which requires clipping with a curved Negus clip and tying with silk (Figure 6.1(e)). The clip is then slowly removed as the tie is thrown and the tie then trimmed. The tonsillar fossa is packed with a tonsil swab while dissection is performed on the opposite side.

Haemostasis is achieved using bipolar diathermy or further ties. Once haemostasis has been achieved, the gag is relaxed for 30 seconds and the mouth reopened. The fossae are inspected for bleeding and dealt with accordingly. Gentle use of the sucker to remove blood from the base of the tongue and under the soft palate is accompanied by the passage of a Jacques suction catheter through the nose to remove a potential 'coroner's' clot from the postnasal space. If not removed, this clot may fall into and obstruct the airway, to be retrieved only later by the coroner. Suction is attached and the catheter gently withdrawn.

The Boyle–Davis gag is relaxed and carefully removed. The endotracheal tube may on occasion herniate into the tongue blade and hence the patient may be inadvertently extubated. This will result in a significant airway compromise and must be avoided.

A survey of the teeth must be performed to document any dental trauma (or loss which will require retrieval of the tooth). The jaw must also be assessed to exclude a temporo-mandibular joint dislocation. It is also essential to confirm that all the tonsil swabs have been removed. Tonsillectomy using coblation has grown in popularity, particularly in paediatric cases where an intracapsular tonsillectomy can be performed, which decreases postoperative pain and can lead to a more rapid recovery. However, it does carry a greater risk of tonsil regrowth that may require further surgery in the future.

POSTOPERATIVE REVIEW AND FOLLOW-UP

Patients undergoing tonsillectomy alone do not require follow-up unless tissue has been sent for histology. Whilst tonsillectomy is routinely performed as a day case procedure, those with obstructive sleep apnoea require overnight observations as an inpatient.

Patients will complain of odonophagia and otalgia, and require regular analgesia for the first postoperative week.

It is essential that patients eat and drink normally as this reduces not only the likelihood of infection but also subsequent secondary bleeding.

POST-TONSILLECTOMY HAEMORRHAGE

This is a potentially life-threatening emergency and should be managed as such. Patients must be assessed in the Emergency Department. Assessment should include the ABC algorithm with early cannulation using wide-bore cannulae. Blood must be taken for a full blood count, clotting screen and group and save.

If the bleeding has spontaneously stopped, patients are admitted for observation.

If bleeding persists behind a tonsillar clot, this should be removed with a Yankauer sucker or Magill's forceps. A tonsil swab or ribbon gauze soaked in 1:5000 adrenaline can be held over the bleeding point and may achieve haemostasis.

If these measures fail, the patient is transferred to theatre for emergency surgical arrest of the haemorrhage. This can be achieved by diathermy or application of a tie. However, the tissue is generally friable in these situations; laying a strip of Surgicel within the tonsillar fossa and over-sewing the anterior and posterior pillars together with a heavy stitch may be required.

REFERENCES

1 Management of sore throat and indications for tonsillectomy, a national clinical guideline (April 2010). Scottish Intercollegiate Guidelines Network, Guideline 117.
2 Lowe D, Van der Meulen J, Cromwell D et al. 2007. Key messages from the National Prospective Tonsillectomy Audit. *Laryngoscope* 117(4): 717–24.

7

ADENOIDECTOMY

Ketan Desai

Indications

- Obstructive sleep apnoea.

- In conjunction with grommet insertion. Adenoidectomy may decrease the risk of further persistent bilateral otitis media with effusion requiring grommets in the future.

PREOPERATIVE REVIEW

One must always be cautious when it comes to operating on small children (<15 kg or <3 years of age) as they have a smaller circulating blood volume and a preoperative group and save sample may be required. One should exclude a personal or familial bleeding tendency and discuss this with a senior colleague if necessary. There is an increase in the vascularity of the adenoidal pad following an upper aero-digestive tract infection, and many surgeons will postpone surgery if there has been a recent episode.

OPERATIVE TECHNIQUE

Two techniques are commonly used for adenoidectomy.

▌ Adenoidal curettage

Once intubated, the patient is placed supine and a shoulder roll is placed under the patient to extend the neck. A headlight is required. The patient is draped, a Boyle–Davis gag inserted and the mouth opened. Once secured with Draffin rods, care should be taken to avoid damage to the teeth and lips and kinking of the endotracheal tube. A finger is inserted into the postnasal space to:

- Confirm the presence of an enlarged adenoidal pad.

- Exclude a pulsatile adenoidal pad (this may actually be an angiofibroma, in which case adenoidectomy is ill advised).
- Exclude the presence of a cleft palate or submucous cleft (an adenoidectomy may result in a nasal voice and nasal regurgitation, and is a contra-indication for curette adenoidectomy).
- To exclude a choanal atresia.
- To sweep the adenoidal pad into the midline.

An adenoidal curette is passed into the postnasal space and the adenoidal pad curetted with firm but gentle pressure. The postnasal space is packed with swabs to achieve haemostasis (several swab changes may be required).

Haemostasis is confirmed by tilting the head forward and inspecting for any bleeding. Further brisk bleeding requires repacking of the postnasal space. Occasionally, suction diathermy or adrenaline soaked packs may be required.

▌ Suction diathermy

This technique has recently gained popularity (Figure 7.1) (1, 2). Evidence suggests that suction diathermy adenoidectomy results in less intra-operative blood loss, less remnant adenoidal tissue and less postoperative nasal regurgitation of food (3).

Once anaesthetized, the patient is placed supine and a shoulder roll inserted in order to extend the neck. A Boyle–Davis mouth gag is inserted and supported with Draffin rods. Jacques catheters are passed through each nostril and the distal ends are drawn out of the oral cavity.

Gentle traction is used to elevate the soft palate. A mirror is inserted into the oral cavity and used to assess the adenoidal pad. If enlarged, suction diathermy is used to cauterize the surface of the pad.

The stem of the suction diathermy is angled to allow access to the adenoidal pad. Great care must be taken to avoid injury to the surrounding structures, including the Eustachian tube cushions. Adequate clearance is gained when both choanae are clearly visible and the posterior pharyngeal wall has a smooth contour.

Complications

- Bleeding.
- Infection.
- *Grisel's syndrome* – atlanto-axial subluxation due to ligamentous laxity as a result of infection.

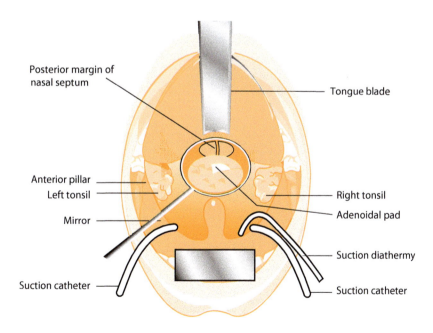

Figure 7.1. Suction diathermy of the adenoidal tissue.

POSTOPERATIVE REVIEW

Patients may develop minor neck stiffness and regular analgesia should be taken for up to a week. Prophylactic oral antibiotics may also be prescribed. If torticollis occurs, this may indicate Grisel's syndrome and the patient should return to hospital.

There is a risk of bleeding for the week following surgery, and relative isolation from other children reduces the risk of viral transmission and the development of secondary haemorrhage. In children this requires one week off school. Should bleeding occur, the patient should attend the Emergency Department immediately.

REFERENCES

1 Hartley BE, Papsin BC, Albert DM. 1998. Suction diathermy adenoidectomy. *Clin Otolaryngol Allied Sci* 23: 308–9.

2 Lo S, Rowe-Jones J. 2006. How we do it: transoral suction diathermy adenoid ablation under direct vision using a 45 degree endoscope. *Clin Otolaryngol* 31: 440–2.

3 Suction Diathermy Adenoidectomy (December 2009). NICE guidance IPG328. www.nice.org.uk/nicemedia/live/12127/46633/46633.pdf.

8 GROMMET INSERTION

Rahul Kanegaonkar

Grommets are tubes placed in the tympanic membrane to ventilate the middle ear space.

Indications

- Persistent bilateral middle ear effusions resulting in >30 dB HL bilateral conductive hearing loss in two or more frequencies for at least three months.
- Recurrent acute otitis media.
- In adults, a unilateral middle ear effusion (combined with a postnasal space examination and biopsy).
- Significant tympanic membrane retraction.
- Mènière's disease.

Current National Institute for Health and Clinical Excellence (NICE) guidelines (CG60 February 2008) recommend direct surgical intervention for otitis media with effusion (OME) in children up to the age of 12 years and who demonstrate a hearing loss due to a persistent middle ear effusion lasting three months or more (1). However, patients must be treated on a case-by-case basis, taking into account their educational progress and speech development. Grommet insertion is not currently recommended for children with Down's syndrome, who are managed with hearing aids.

PATIENT INFORMATION AND CONSENT

The rationale for grommet insertion and alternative treatment with hearing aids should be discussed.

Grommets remain in place for an average of 18 months in the paediatric age group. In 30% of children, middle ear effusions recur once the grommets have extruded.

OPERATIVE PROCEDURE

In children and in most adults, this procedure is performed under general anaesthetic.

The anaesthetized patient is positioned supine and the head rotated away from the operator, who is seated. A perforated ear drape is placed over the ear. The largest aural speculum that comfortably fits in the canal is used. This is held

with the non-dominant hand and the microscope focused to provide a clear image of the tympanic membrane (Figure 8.1(a)). Any wax is removed using a Jobson–Horne probe, crocodile forceps or a Zoellner sucker. Care must be taken not to traumatize the canal mucosa. If bleeding does occur, a cotton wool pledget soaked in 1:10,000 adrenaline provides haemostasis.

The anteroinferior quadrant is identified and a myringotome used to make a radial incision from the umbo towards the annulus (Figure 8.1(b)). As the incision is performed, a note is made of the presence of an effusion and its appearance (Figure 8.1(c)). This is removed gently with suction using a fine end attached to a Zoellner sucker.

Forceps are used to grasp the grommet at either its rim or heel (Figure 8.1(e), (f)). Once firmly grasped, the long axis of the grommet should be in line with the long axis of the forceps (Figure 8.1(g)).

The grommet is advanced such that its toe is inserted into the myringotomy incision. Gentle pressure applied at the heel of the grommet with a needle is usually required to push the grommet into place (Figure 8.1(h)).

A grommet inadvertently pushed into the middle ear may be retrieved by a senior colleague.

The use of topical ear drops immediately following grommet insertion has gained popularity and may reduce the incidence of grommet blockage (2).

Complications

- Recurrent ear infections, occasionally requiring removal of the grommet.
- Persistent perforation (1%–2%); patients may require a myringoplasty in order to close the perforation (3).

Figure 8.1. Grommet insertion.

POSTOPERATIVE REVIEW AND FOLLOW-UP

Many surgeons advise that the ears are kept absolutely dry for at least 2 weeks after the procedure. Patients may be allowed to swim with grommets in place several weeks after insertion, unless they suffer recurrent ear infections.

Patients are reviewed after 12 weeks with repeat audiometry.

REFERENCES

1 Surgical management of children with otitis media with effusion (OME) (February 2008). NICE clinical guidance CG60. Available at: guidance.nice.org.uk/CG60.

2 Arya AK, Rea PA, Robinson PJ. 2004. The use of perioperative Sofradex eardrops in preventing tympanostomy tube blockage: a prospective double-blinded randomized-controlled trial. *Clin Otolaryngol Allied Sci* 29: 598–601.

3 Lous J, Burton MJ, Felding JU et al. 2005. Grommets (ventilation tubes) for hearing loss associated with otitis media with effusion in children. *Cochrane Database Syst Rev* 25(1): CD001801.

SEPTOPLASTY

Joanne Rimmer

Nasal obstruction due to a deviated nasal septum was previously corrected by submucous resection (SMR). This involves excising much of the septal cartilage and bone, irrespective of the deviation, leaving an 'L-strut' of dorsal and caudal septum for support. This procedure has given way to septoplasty, which involves resection of as little septal cartilage and bone as possible (Figure 9.1), specifically at areas of deviation, and aims to reposition the septum in the midline (1). This retains more septal support, and reduces the risk of postoperative septal perforation (2).

Indications

- Nasal obstruction secondary to a deviated nasal septum. Patient selection is paramount. Those with nasal obstruction due to septal deviation alone have an excellent outcome (3). If the obstruction is mainly due to mucosal disease (e.g. allergic rhinitis) then the results are often less satisfactory (4).
- Cosmetic correction of a deviated nose as part of a septorhinoplasty. If there is severe deviation of the mid- and lower thirds of the nose, such

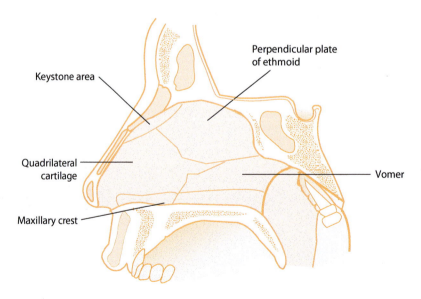

Figure 9.1. The nasal septum.

as in the twisted nose, then an extracorporeal septoplasty technique may be required (5).

- To facilitate the use of nasal continuous positive airway pressure (CPAP) devices in obstructive sleep apnoea (OSA).
- Access for endoscopic sinonasal or skull base procedures.
- In the management of epistaxis where a deviated septum prevents adequate nasal packing.
- To harvest septal cartilage for use as an autograft.

OPERATIVE PROCEDURE

An appropriately informed, consented and anaesthetized patient is positioned supine, head up or in a beach chair position, with a head ring for support. Topical nasal preparations such as Moffett's solution (a variable mixture of cocaine, adrenaline, normal saline and sodium bicarbonate) (6) or co-phenylcaine spray (5% lidocaine and 0.5% phenylephrine) may be instilled into the nose to improve the surgical field. The patient's eyes are taped closed or lubricating ointment is instilled. The surgeon wears a headlight, although the procedure may be performed endoscopically (7).

Skin preparation is not routinely used. The patient is draped with a head towel and the face is exposed from the eyebrows to upper lip. The nasal cavities and septal deviation are then assessed using a Killian's or Cottle's nasal speculum. It is important to identify the side and site of the deviation, and relate this to the patient's obstructive symptoms (Figure 9.2).

A short nasal speculum is held with one blade on either side of the caudal edge of the quadrilateral cartilage, and both sides of the septum are infiltrated with a solution of 2% lidocaine with 1:80,000 adrenaline using a dental syringe (Figure 9.3(a)). The mucoperichondrium should blanche following infiltration, which aids haemostasis.

A number 15 scalpel blade is used to incise the mucoperichondrium down to cartilage (Figure 9.3(b)). This incision can be placed along the caudal edge of the quadrilateral cartilage at the septocolumellar junction (hemitransfixion incision) or approximately 0.5 cm behind the

Compensatory hypertrophy of the right inferior turbinate

Figure 9.2. Septal deviation to the left.

mucocutaneous junction (Killian's incision) (Figure 9.4). It is often easier to find the correct plane of dissection using a Killian's incision, but it is difficult to address very caudal septal deviations though this incision. The incision is usually made on the left (for a right-handed surgeon), but in certain cases (e.g. caudal septal dislocation to the right) the surgeon may elect to make the incision on the right.

It is important to find the correct plane for dissection; this is subperichondrial, between the cartilage and the perichondrium. It is all too easy to dissect the plane between perichondrium

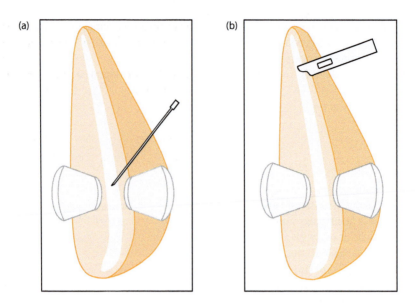

Figure 9.3. Infiltration of the septal mucosa (a) before an incision is made (b).

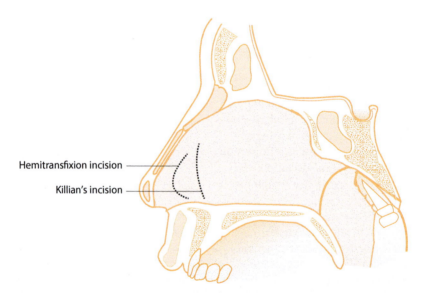

Figure 9.4. Incisions for a septoplasty. A hemitransfixion incision is made along the caudal (anterior) edge of the septum, whilst a Killian's incision is made 0.5 cm posterior to the mucocutaneous junction.

and mucosa in error. Perichondrium has a pale pink appearance due to its blood supply, whereas septal cartilage has a shiny white/pale blue colour. If a hemitransfixion incision has been made, sharp pointed scissors are helpful initially as the mucopericondrium is tethered anteriorly due to McGilligan's fibres. The shortest nasal speculum may be pressed firmly into the incision against the cartilage to assist dissection (Figure 9.5).

Once the plane has been identified, insert a Freer elevator between the cartilage and mucoperichondrium and raise the mucoperichondrial flap carefully along the full

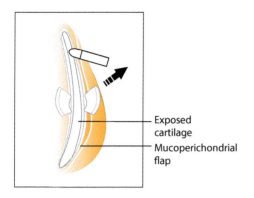

Figure 9.5. A Freer elevator is used to dissect the mucoperichondrium from septal cartilage.

length of the septum. It is often easier to elevate the flap superiorly first, where it is less adherent, and continue inferiorly and posteriorly with gentle sweeping movements.

Care must be taken not to tear the flap, which can be particularly difficult over spurs or fracture lines. Another area of difficulty is at the junction of the septal cartilage and maxillary crest bone inferiorly, as the mucoperiosteum overlying the latter is more tightly adherent than the mucoperichondrium is to the quadrilateral cartilage, and the two are not in continuity. It can be helpful to raise the mucoperiostium more posteriorly over the vomer first, and then continue the dissection anteriorly with a hockey stick dissector.

The procedure from this point is determined by the site and extent of the deviation. If the quadrilateral cartilage is attached to a deviated bony septum, incise the osseochondral junction to release it posteriorly. The area of cartilaginous deviation may be amenable to resection, in which case the quadrilateral cartilage is fully incised at the appropriate point (often the most deviated part), and then a partial contralateral flap is elevated posteriorly from the transcartilaginous incision to allow removal of the intervening piece of cartilage or bone (Figure 9.6(a–c)). If removing bony septum is required, scissors or through-cutting forceps (e.g. Jansen-Middleton forceps) should be used in order to avoid twisting the perpendicular plate of the ethmoid (PPE), as there is a theoretical risk of skull base fracture at the cribriform plate with subsequent cerebrospinal fluid (CSF) leak.

When removing quadrilateral cartilage, it is vital to understand the major areas of support that should not be resected. The most important is the keystone area (Figure 9.1); this is the junction of the quadrilateral cartilage, PPE, nasal bones and upper lateral cartilages. The cartilage and bone should not be completely separated at this point to avoid dorsal collapse. It is advisable to leave at least 1 cm dorsal and caudal struts of septal cartilage for support, although in practice one would aim to leave much more cartilage in place if feasible. Bony spurs inferiorly may be resected using a fishtail gouge. The septal cartilage may

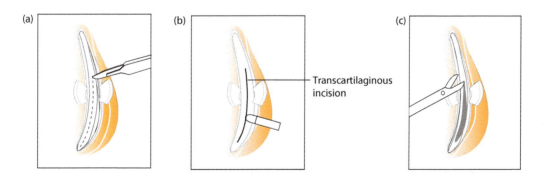

Figure 9.6. An incision is made through the septal cartilage (a). A Freer elevator is passed through the incision and the mucoperichondrium elevated off the cartilage on the contralateral side (b). Turbinectomy scissors may be used to excise the deviated cartilage (c).

be incised (often along fracture lines) in order to help repositioning, and various scoring, cutting and suturing techniques have been described, particularly to address the most difficult problem of caudal deviation (8,9).

It is sometimes necessary to elevate a complete contralateral mucoperichondrial flap, in which case the plane can be followed over the caudal edge of the quadrilateral cartilage onto the right side and dissected as above. This is usually only necessary in severe and/or caudal deviations, and is avoided if possible to reduce the risk of septal perforation.

Once the deviation has been corrected, the incision is closed with a 4/0 or 5/0 absorbable suture. The same suture should be used to 'quilt' the septum with continuous through-and-through mattress sutures. This reduces the risk of septal haematoma formation by closing the dead space (Figure 9.7). Nasal packing is not routinely inserted.

Figure 9.7. Continuous quilting suture of the nasal septum, secured anteriorly.

POSTOPERATIVE REVIEW

The patient can be discharged the same day or the next day according to local protocol. Discharge medication should include analgesia and nasal douches. Patients are advised to take 7–14 days off work, avoid nose-blowing for one week and avoid heavy lifting or strenuous exercise for two weeks. Follow-up should be after three months.

Complications

- *Bleeding* – Some oozing is normal but heavy epistaxis requires return to hospital and may warrant nasal packing. If a septal haematoma develops it will require draining and packing.
- *Infection*.

- *Ongoing symptoms* – Either related to persistent/recurrent deviation as septal cartilage has 'memory', or to concurrent mucosal disease.
- *Septal perforation* – Usually asymptomatic, but may cause crusting, bleeding or whistling.
- *Cosmetic change* – Significant collapse (saddle nose) is rare, but subtle changes are probably underrecognised by patients and surgeons.

REFERENCES
1 Fettman N, Sanford T, Sindwani R. 2009. Surgical management of the deviated septum: Techniques in septoplasty. *Otolaryngologic Clin N Am* 42: 241–52.

2 Goode RL, Smith LF. 2001. Nasal septoplasty and submucous resection. In: *Atlas of Head & Neck Surgery – Otolaryngology*. 2nd ed. p. 462–4. Lippincott Williams & Wilkins, Philadelphia.

3 Moore M, Eccles R. 2011. Objective evidence for the efficacy of surgical management of the deviated septum as treatment for chronic nasal obstruction: A systematic review. *Clin Otolaryngol* 36: 106–13.

4 Karatzanis AD, Fragiadakis G, Moshandrea J, Zenk J, Iro H, Velegrakis GA. 2009. Septoplasty outcome in patients with and without allergic rhinitis. *Rhinology* 47: 444–9.

5 Wu PS, Hamilton GS 3rd. 2016. Extracorporeal septoplasty: External and endonasal techniques. *Facial Plast Surg* 32: 22–8.

6 Benjamin E, Wong DKK, Choa D. 2004. 'Moffett's' solution: A review of the evidence and scientific basis for the topical preparation of the nose. *Clin Otolaryngol* 29: 582–7.

7 Champagne C, Ballivet de Régloix S, Genestier L, Crambert A, Maurin O, Pons Y. 2016. Endoscopic vs. conventional septoplasty: A review of the literature. *Eur Ann Otorhinolaryngol Head Neck Dis* 133: 43–6.

8 Jang YJ, Yeo NK, Wang JH. 2009. Cutting and suture technique of the caudal septal cartilage for the management of caudal septal deviation. *Archiv Otolaryngol Head Neck Surg* 135: 1256–60.

9 Kenyon GS, Kalan A, Jones NS. 2002. Columelloplasty: A new suture technique to correct caudal septal cartilage dislocation. *Clin Otolaryngol* 27: 188–91.

10 SEPTORHINOPLASTY

Joanne Rimmer

There are numerous techniques involved in rhinoplasty surgery which are beyond the scope of this book. Briefly, it can be divided into the endonasal (closed) approach and the external (open) approach (1, 2). The endonasal approach is discussed here.

Indications

- *Functional* – To correct nasal obstruction that would not be otherwise successfully managed with simple septoplasty alone.
- Cosmetic correction of a deviated nose (±septum).

PREOPERATIVE REVIEW

Patient selection in rhinoplasty is paramount; expectations must be realistic. Standard preoperative photographs are required in lateral, frontal, oblique, bird's eye and basal views.

OPERATIVE PROCEDURE

An appropriately informed, consented and anaesthetized patient should be positioned supine or in a beach chair position, head up, with a head ring for support. Topical nasal preparations such as Moffett's solution (a variable mixture of cocaine, adrenaline, normal saline and sodium bicarbonate) or co-phenylcaine spray (5% lidocaine and 0.5% phenylephrine) may be instilled into the nose to improve the surgical field. The patient's eyes are taped closed (over the lateral aspect only) or lubricating ointment is instilled. A headlight is worn, although overhead operating lights may be used in the external approach.

Skin preparation is used around the nose. The patient is draped with a head towel so that the face is exposed from eyebrows to upper lip.

The septum is infiltrated with 2% lidocaine with 1:80,000 adrenaline as for a septoplasty (Chapter 9). Infiltration is continued superiorly in the nasal vestibules, along the lines of intercartilaginous incisions (Figure 10.1). It is continued into the soft tissue overlying the dorsum of the nose, and particularly at the incision sites for external lateral osteotomies. The nasal hairs are removed with a scalpel blade or short curved scissors.

Septoplasty is performed via a left hemitransfixion incision as described in Chapter 9. Once this is completed, bilateral intercartilaginous incisions are made between the upper and lower lateral cartilages (Figure 10.1). The groove between the cartilages is best displayed using an alar retractor with external pressure from the surgeon's middle finger.

Upper lateral cartilage
Lower lateral cartilage
Line of an intercartilaginous incision

Figure 10.1. Intercartilaginous incision.

Care is taken not to incise the cartilages themselves. On the left, the incision is continued caudally into the hemitransfixion incision. On the right, the incision is extended caudally and through into the left hemitransfixion incision to complete a full transfixion incision, although this does not need to extend completely to the base of the columella.

The dorsal nasal skin and soft tissue envelope is then degloved with a number 15 scalpel blade or curved scissors, taking care not to buttonhole the skin by staying on cartilage/bone. The skin should be freed superiorly to the nasion and approximately halfway down the lateral walls to allow adequate visualization of the nasal dorsum with an Aufricht retractor and the scissors to pass freely from one side of the nose to the other. Release the procerus muscle at the nasion using a periostial elevator.

A dorsal hump can be removed with a 6–8 mm osteotome, taking care not to buttonhole the skin at either side (Figure 10.2). The dorsum should then be rasped smooth.

Bilateral external lateral osteotomies are performed with a 2 mm osteotome, via two small stab incisions made with a number 11 scalpel blade on either side of the nose. The line of the osteotomy is 'postage-stamped' with multiple small osteotomies along the lines shown in Figure 10.3. The assistant stabilizes the patient's head while the surgeon employs the mallet. Lateral

Figure 10.2. An osteotome may be used to remove a dorsal hump once the overlying soft tissue envelope has been lifted. The line of the osteotomy is illustrated.

Figure 10.3. Medial and lateral osteotomy.

osteotomies may also be performed endonasally via a stab incision just anterior to the head of the inferior turbinate. Bilateral medial osteotomies are performed internally, using a 4–6 mm osteotome via the nasal cavity or through the intercartilaginous incision. It should be positioned perpendicular to the caudal end of the nasal bone, just lateral to the septum. The line of the osteotomy is shown in Figure 10.3. The assistant gently taps with the mallet, while the surgeon palpates the edge of the osteotome with the second hand to ensure its position and to prevent buttonholing the skin. Firm digital pressure is used to reposition the bones appropriately.

In more complex cases, tip sutures or grafts may be required; these are often better undertaken via an external approach.

The incisions are closed with a 4/0 or 5/0 absorbable suture. The same suture should be used to 'quilt' the septum with through-and-through mattress sutures to reduce the risk of septal haematoma formation by closing the dead space as for standard septoplasty. Steristrips are applied over the dorsum and to support the tip, and a triangular plaster of Paris is placed over these. Nasal packing is not routinely inserted.

POSTOPERATIVE REVIEW

The patient can be discharged the same day or the next day according to local protocol. Discharge medication should include analgesia. Patients are advised to take 10–14 days off work, avoid nose-blowing for one week and avoid heavy lifting or strenuous exercise for two weeks. They are warned to expect periorbital bruising and swelling. Initial follow-up is after 7–10 days for removal of the plaster, after which patients can begin to douche the nose.

Complications

- *Bleeding* – Some oozing is normal but heavy epistaxis requires return to hospital and may warrant nasal packing. If a septal haematoma develops it will require draining and packing.
- *Infection*.

- *Ongoing obstructive symptoms* – Either related to persistent/recurrent deviation as septal cartilage has 'memory', or to concurrent mucosal disease.
- *Septal perforation* – Usually asymptomatic but may cause crusting, bleeding or whistling.
- *Ongoing cosmetic concerns* – Patients should be advised of a 5%–10% revision rate following primary rhinoplasty surgery.

REFERENCES
1 Daniel RK. 2010. *Mastering Rhinoplasty*. 2nd ed. Springer-Verlag, Berlin Heidelberg.
2 Nolst Trenite GJ. 2005. *Rhinoplasty: A Practical Guide to Functional and Aesthetic Surgery of the Nose*. 3rd ed. Kugler Publications, The Hague.

11 TURBINATE SURGERY

Joanne Rimmer

Indications

- Nasal obstruction secondary to inferior turbinate (IT) hypertrophy refractory to medical treatment.

OPERATIVE PROCEDURE

There is an ever-increasing number of methods to reduce ITs, and a Cochrane review found no high quality evidence for any one technique over another (1). All are performed in an appropriately informed, consented and anaesthetized patient positioned supine or in a beach chair position, head up, with a head ring for support. Topical nasal preparations such as Moffett's solution (a variable mixture of cocaine, adrenaline, normal saline and sodium bicarbonate) or co-phenylcaine spray (5% lidocaine and 0.5% phenylephrine) may be instilled into the nose to improve the surgical field. A headlight may be worn by the surgeon or a rigid Hopkins rod used for endoscopic techniques. The patient's eyes are taped closed. Skin preparation is not routinely used. The patient is draped with a head towel with the nose exposed.

▌ Outfracture of inferior turbinate

A Hill' elevator is used to first infracture (medialize) the IT and then outfracture (lateralize) it (Figure 11.1).

Figure 11.1. Outfracture of the right inferior turbinate.

▌ Radiofrequency or coblation turbinoplasty

A Thudichum's speculum is used to allow visualization of the IT. A radiofrequency or coblation turbinate probe, both of which are commercially available, is inserted into the inferior turbinate soft tissue, medial to the bone, and then activated. Three passes are generally performed, superiorly, inferiorly, and at the

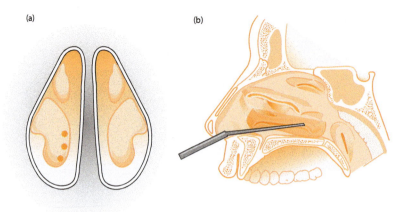

Figure 11.2. Radiofrequency turbinoplasty. (a) Points of turbinate probe contact. (b) Probe in situ.

midpoint of the IT (Figure 11.2). The specific techniques vary depending to the device used, but the radiofrequency energy is transmitted to the submucosal soft tissue of the IT, ablating it, with a subsequent reduction in the size of the IT (2, 3).

A similar technique using a submucosal monopolar diathermy needle has been employed for many years, but it tends to cause significant postoperative crusting in the nose and the results are less predictable than newer techniques used.

▌ Inferior turbinoplasty

Multiple methods and instruments are used to remove the IT soft tissue and bone whilst preserving the medial mucosa, either with a head light or endoscopically. In all cases, the IT is infiltrated with 2% lidocaine with 1:80,000 adrenaline using a dental syringe. In the cold steel technique, a scalpel blade is used to make a stab incision over the anterior end of the IT bone. A Freer elevator is used to elevate the medial mucosa off the bone approximately one-half to two-thirds along the length of the IT. This flap is then detached inferiorly using turbinectomy scissors which are then used to remove the turbinate bone and lateral soft tissue. The mucosal flap is then replaced and can be supported with a length of absorbable packing. This can be done with a headlight or endoscopically, and the microdebrider

can be used to reduce the soft tissue inferiorly and laterally prior to elevation of the medial mucosal flap (4). A specific turbinoplasty microdebrider attachment is also available, which is inserted through a stab incision as above and allows powered removal of IT bone and soft tissue (5).

Figure 11.3. Turbinectomy. Care must be taken to avoid damage to the nasolacrimal duct.

■ Turbinectomy

This may be done using a headlight or endoscope. The IT is first infractured as above, then turbinectomy scissors are used to trim it along its inferomedial aspect (Figure 11.3).

A length of absorbable packing may be placed along the cut surface. If there is significant bleeding a nasal tampon may be required, in which case the patient should be kept overnight and the pack removed the following morning.

POSTOPERATIVE REVIEW

The patient can be discharged the same day or the next day according to local protocol. Discharge medication includes analgesia and nasal douche; regular intranasal steroid treatment for rhinitis should be recommenced after a few days. Patients are advised to take one week off work and to avoid nose-blowing for one week and heavy lifting or strenuous exercise for two weeks. Follow-up may be arranged.

Complications

- *Bleeding* – This may be torrential and patients should be warned of the potential need for a blood transfusion. The risk is higher with turbinectomy than turbinoplasty.
- *Nasal crusting* – Turbinectomy leaves a large raw area, unlike turbinoplasty; diathermy can also cause crusting.
- *Adhesions* – Between the IT and septum.
- *Empty nose syndrome* – Excessive removal of IT tissue has been implicated in worsening symptoms of obstruction, possibly due to a loss of sensation of nasal airflow; hence, the newer turbinoplasty procedures do not remove the medial mucosa.

- *Ongoing/recurrent symptoms* – Any benefit may be temporary, and ongoing medical treatment of rhinitis may be required postoperatively.

REFERENCES

1 Jose J, Coatesworth AP. 2010. Inferior turbinate surgery for nasal obstruction in allergic rhinitis after failed medical management. *Cochrane Database Syst Rev* 8: CD005235.
2 Benjamin E, Wong DKK, Choa D. 2004. 'Moffett's' solution: A review of the evidence and scientific basis for the topical preparation.
3 Lin HC, Lin PW, Friedman M, Chang HW, Su YY, Chen YJ, Pulver TM. 2010. Long-term results of radiofrequency turbinoplasty for allergic rhinitis refractory to medical therapy. *Archiv Otolaryngol Head Neck Surg* 136: 892–5.
4 Di Rienzo Businco L, Di Rienzo Businco A, Lauriello M. 2010. Comparative study on the effectiveness of coblation-assisted turbinoplasty in allergic rhinitis. *Rhinology* 48: 174–8.
5 Barham HP, Knisely A, Harvey RJ, Sacks R. 2015. How I do it: medial flap inferior turbinoplasty. *Am J Rhinol Allergy* 29: 314–5.

12 ENDOSCOPIC SINUS SURGERY (ESS)

Joanne Rimmer

Also referred to as 'functional endoscopic sinus surgery' (FESS), the aim of endoscopic sinus surgery (ESS) is to improve the function of the paranasal sinuses and/or to allow better instillation of topical medication. Mucosal stripping is avoided and the natural sinus ostia are opened whenever possible. There are also a number of extended applications of ESS, including those listed below (1).

Indications

- Chronic rhinosinusitis with or without nasal polyps, refractory to maximum medical treatment.
- Recurrent acute rhinosinusitis.
- Complications of acute rhinosinusitis.
- Mucocoele.
- Sinonasal tumour excision.
- Orbital or optic nerve decompression.
- Endoscopic repair of CSF leak.
- Endoscopic approach to pituitary/anterior skull base lesions.

PREOPERATIVE REVIEW

A CT scan of the sinuses is mandatory, and should be available at the time of surgery. This must be reviewed pre-operatively by the surgeon to evaluate the extent of disease, any previous surgery or bony loss, and any anatomical variants (2).

OPERATIVE PROCEDURE

An appropriately informed, consented and anaesthetized patient should be positioned supine, head up or in a beach chair position, with a head ring for support. Topical nasal preparations such as Moffett's solution (a variable mixture of cocaine, adrenaline, normal saline and sodium bicarbonate) or dilute adrenaline are instilled into the nose to improve the surgical field. The patient's eyes are not taped or covered, but lubricating ointment is instilled. This allows immediate identification of any orbital movement or bleeding, and for the eye to be balloted while observing the lateral nasal wall for any evidence of movement (suggesting a dehiscent lamina papyracea). Skin preparation is not routinely used. The patient is draped with a head towel, exposing the nose and eyes.

A 0° rigid Hopkins rod endoscope is used to inspect the nasal cavities bilaterally using the three-pass technique (see Chapter 2). The first pass is along the floor of the nose to the postnasal space, assessing the inferior meatus (Figure 12.1). The second is into the middle meatus (Figure 12.2), and the third into the superior meatus and olfactory niche; the sphenoid ostium may be identified during this pass. Important landmarks to note are the septum, inferior and middle turbinates, and the posterior choana.

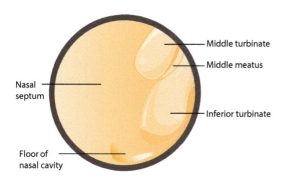

Figure 12.1 View of first pass along the floor of the left nasal cavity.

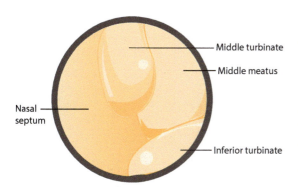

Figure 12.2 The second pass allows access to the middle meatus (left).

At this point, it is helpful to insert neuropatties or ribbon gauze soaked in 1:10,000 adrenaline into the middle meatus, using a Freer elevator for accurate positioning. This will provide further decongestion and vasoconstriction to improve the surgical field.

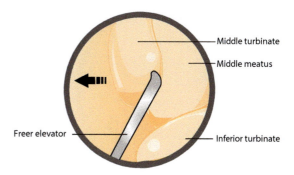

Figure 12.3 Gentle medialization of the left middle turbinate to access the middle meatus.

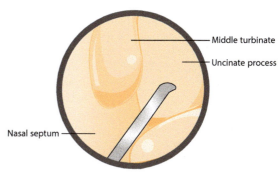

Figure 12.4 Palpation of the free posterior edge of the uncinate process with a Freer elevator.

The middle turbinate should not be forcefully medialized as this risks skull base fracture with cerebrospinal fluid (CSF) leak. It can be gently medialized, but if very large and obstructing, then a wedge can be removed from the anterior end with a through cutting punch whilst preserving the majority as an anatomical landmark (Figure 12.3).

The uncinate process is palpated with a Freer elevator to identify its free posterior border and its anterior attachment (Figure 12.4).

An uncinectomy is performed to expose the natural ostium of the maxillary sinus, with either an anterograde (anterior to posterior) or retrograde (posterior to anterior) technique. In the anterograde method, the Freer elevator or a sickle knife is used to incise along the anterior attachment of the uncinate process from inferior

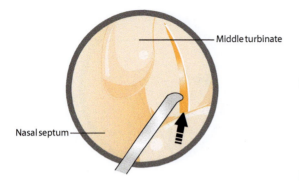

Figure 12.5 Incision along the anterior attachment of the uncinate process.

Figure 12.7 View of the left middle meatal antrostomy and ethmoid bulla after removal of the uncinate process.

to superior (Figure 12.5). Care should be taken not to enter the orbit with this incision.

Endoscopic scissors are used to cut through the remaining superior and inferior attachments of the uncinate process, or straight Blakesley–Wilde forceps can be used with a twisting motion to avoid tearing the mucosa (Figure 12.6).

The retrograde technique is said to reduce the risk of orbital penetration. A backbiting forceps is placed behind the free posterior edge of the uncinate process at its most inferior point and the uncinate is detached inferiorly. A 45° angled through-cutter is then used to remove it along its anterior attachment.

Once the uncinectomy is complete, the natural maxillary ostium should be visible and the ethmoid bulla will also be in view (Figure 12.7).

A curved sucker may be passed into the maxillary sinus to remove any mucus or pus. The antrostomy may be widened if necessary using a backbiting forceps or the microdebrider. The ethmoid bulla is opened using 45° angled Blakesley–Wilde forceps or a small curette behind its inferior edge.

The anterior ethmoids are opened with a curette or Blakesely–Wilde forceps (Figure 12.8), as are the posterior ethmoids, if indicated. Appropriately trained and experienced surgeons may perform sphenoid sinus and frontal recess surgery, as required.

If bleeding is minimal then no packing is required. Depending on the surgeon's preference and the amount of bleeding, packing may be inserted into the middle meatus, in the form of adrenaline-soaked ribbon gauze or newer absorbable packing materials.

Figure 12.6 Removal of the left uncinate process.

Figure 12.8 Opening of the left anterior ethmoid cells.

If non-absorbable nasal packing is inserted, it can be removed in recovery, on the ward or the next morning depending on the amount of oozing. The patient may be discharged the same day or the next day as per local protocol. Discharge medication can include analgesics, oral and/or topical nasal steroids and nasal douche. Antibiotics may be given. Patients are advised to avoid nose-blowing for one week and have 7–14 days off work, avoid heavy lifting or strenuous exercise during this time. Follow-up should be after two weeks to allow for outpatient decrusting of the nasal cavities.

Complications

- *Bleeding* – Some oozing is normal but heavy epistaxis may warrant nasal packing or, rarely, return to theatre. Perioperative haemorrhage occurs in approximately 5% of cases, with significant postoperative bleeding in less than 1% (3).
- *Infection*.
- *Nasal crusting* – This is minimized with regular douching and early outpatient review.
- *Adhesions* – These usually occur between the middle turbinate and the lateral nasal wall, but can occur between the inferior turbinate and the septum if traumatized during surgery.
- *Recurrent symptoms* – It is important that patients are made aware that ESS not a cure

for the underlying disease process (e.g. chronic rhinosinusitis with or without nasal polyps), and that symptoms can recur. They are, therefore, advised to continue long-term treatment with intranasal steroids and douche after surgery.

- *Orbital injury or bleeding* – This occurs in approximately 0.2% of cases (3).
- *CSF leak* – This occurs in approximately 0.06% of cases (3).

REFERENCES

1 Wormald P-J. 2005. *Endoscopic Sinus Surgery: Anatomy, Three-Dimensional Reconstruction, and Surgical Technique*. Thieme Medical Publishers, New York.

2 Lund VJ, Stammberger H, Fokkens WJ et al. 2004. European position paper on the anatomical terminology of the internal nose and paranasal sinuses. *Rhinology* 50(Suppl. 24): 1–34.

3 Hopkins C, Browne JP, Slack R, Lund VJ, Topham J, Reeves BC, Copley LP, Brown P, van der Meulen JH. 2006. Complications of surgery for nasal polyposis and chronic rhinosinusitis: the results of a national audit in England and Wales. *Laryngoscope* 116: 1494–9.

13 NASAL POLYPECTOMY

Joanne Rimmer

Indications

● Nasal polyposis causing obstructive symptoms despite maximum medical management.

● Histological identification in cases of unilateral polyps.

PREOPERATIVE REVIEW

As nasal polypectomy is now invariably performed as an endoscopic procedure, a CT scan of the sinuses is mandatory. This should be available at the time of surgery and should be reviewed pre-operatively by the surgeon, to evaluate the extent of disease, any previous surgery or bony loss and any anatomical variants (1). Nasal polypectomy is commonly combined with endoscopic sinus surgery (ESS), as there is evidence that even limited ESS in addition to polypectomy can reduce revision rates over a 5-year period (2).

OPERATIVE PROCEDURE

An appropriately informed, consented and anaesthetized patient should be positioned supine, head up or in a beach chair position, with a head ring for support. Topical nasal preparations such as Moffett's solution (a variable mixture of cocaine, adrenaline, normal saline and sodium bicarbonate) or co-phenylcaine spray (5% lidocaine and 0.5% phenylephrine) are instilled into the nose to improve the surgical field, if the extent of polyposis allows. The patient's eyes are not taped or covered, but lubricating ointment is instilled. This allows immediate identification of any orbital bleeding. Skin preparation is not routinely used. The patient is draped with a head towel, exposing the nose and eyes.

A 0° rigid Hopkins rod endoscope is used to inspect the nasal cavities bilaterally. Representative biopsies are taken from both sides. Neuropatties or ribbon gauze soaked in 1:10,000 adrenaline are inserted bilaterally for further decongestion and vasoconstriction.

Polyps are commonly removed using powered instrumentation in the form of a microdebrider. This instrument consists of an oscillating cutting blade within a sheath, attached to irrigation and suction. Care must be taken to ensure that the tip of the instrument can be seen at all times to avoid damage to adjacent structures. Alternatively, grasping instruments such as Blakesley–Wilde forceps are used; 45° angled forceps may be useful for more complete clearance superiorly. Care must be taken not to exert too much force when removing tissue; gentle pressure or a twisting motion should be sufficient.

If bleeding is minimal then no packing is required. Depending on the surgeon's preference and the amount of bleeding, packing may be inserted in the form of adrenaline-soaked ribbon gauze or newer absorbable packing materials, or more rarely a nasal tampon.

POSTOPERATIVE REVIEW

If non-absorbable nasal packing is inserted, it can be removed in recovery, on the ward or the next morning, depending on the amount of oozing. The patient may be discharged the same day or the next day as per local protocol. Discharge medication can include analgesics, oral and/or topical nasal steroids and nasal douche. Antibiotics may be given. Patients are advised to avoid nose-blowing for one week and have 7–14 days off work, avoiding heavy lifting or strenuous exercise during this time. Follow-up should be after two weeks to allow for outpatient decrusting of the nasal cavities.

Complications

- *Bleeding* – Some oozing is normal, but heavy epistaxis may warrant nasal packing or rarely return to theatre.
- *Infection.*
- *Recurrent symptoms/polyps* – It is important to make patients aware that polypectomy is not a cure for the underlying disease process, and that polyps tend to recur. They are, therefore, advised to continue long-term treatment with intranasal steroids and douche after surgery.
- *Persistent anosmia* – Surgical polypectomy does not guarantee the return of a sense of smell, and may even reduce it.
- *Orbital injury or bleeding* – This is unlikely in the absence of formal ESS, but the lamina papyracea may be dehiscent in nasal polyposis.
- *Cerebrospinal fluid (CSF) leak* – Again, this is unlikely in the absence of formal ESS, but polyp removal in the region of the olfactory niche may damage the cribriform plate.

REFERENCES

1 Lund VJ, Stammberger H, Fokkens WJ et al. 2004. European position paper on the anatomical terminology of the internal nose and paranasal sinuses. *Rhinology* 50(Suppl. 24): 1–34.
2 Hopkins C, Slack R, Lund V, Brown P, Copley L, Browne J. 2009. Long-term outcomes from the English national comparative audit of surgery for nasal polyposis and chronic rhinosinusitis. *Laryngoscope* 119: 2459–65.

14 TYMPANOPLASTY

Neil Donnelly and Olivia Kenyon

DEFINITION

Tympanoplasty is the term used for the surgical eradication of middle ear disease and the restoration of middle ear function, including the reconstruction of the tympanic membrane and ossicular chain (ossiculoplasty).

Historically, Wullstein described five types of tympanoplasty (1):

Type 1 – Myringoplasty – closure of a tympanic membrane perforation.

Type 2 – Reconstruction of the tympanic membrane over the malleus remnant and long process of incus.

Type 3 – Reconstruction of the tympanic membrane over the head of the stapes.

Type 4 – Reconstruction of the tympanic membrane over the round window.

Type 5 – Reconstruction of the tympanic membrane over an artificial fenestration in the basal turn of the cochlea.

Type 6 – Reconstruction of the tympanic membrane over an artificial fenestration in the horizontal semicircular canal.

Only two of these remain relevant today.

Type I tympanoplasty describes the reconstruction of the tympanic membrane in the presence of an intact and mobile ossicular chain. This procedure is synonymous with the term myringoplasty.

Type III tympanoplasty describes the reconstruction performed when the incus and malleus have been removed or eroded by disease. The tympanic membrane is reconstructed to lie on the stapes head to create a columella effect or myringostapediopexy. The same principle is applied with some ossiculoplasty procedures, where the stapes superstructure or footplate is in contact with the reconstructed tympanic membrane via a prosthesis.

Indications

- Recurrent ear infection.
- Hearing loss.
- To 'waterproof' the ear.

The main indications for tympanoplasty are chronic secretory otitis media, either mucosal (tympanic membrane perforation) or with cholesteatoma, and the surgical management of pars tensa retraction pockets. These conditions often result in ear discharge (otorrhoea), conductive hearing loss, and the social inconvenience of being unable to get the ear wet.

PREOPERATIVE ASSESSMENT

▌ History

Establish the nature of the symptoms and the impact that these have on the patients' quality of life; this will help when counseling them. Does the ear discharge? How often? Is it painful?

Is there any subjective hearing loss? Is there any associated vertigo or tinnitus? What about the other ear? Is there any other relevant ENT history?

▌ Examination

Document the position (central or marginal) and size of the perforation. Is there an associated cholesteatoma? Describe the status of the middle ear (dry or infected). Is it possible to comment on the state of the ossicular chain?

If there is a pars tensa retraction pocket, it is helpful to use the descriptive Sade classification (See Table 14.1). Document the state of the contralateral ear.

Table 14.1. Sade classification (2).

Grade	Description
1	Mild retraction of pars tensa
2	Retraction touching the incus or stapes
3	Retraction touching the promontory
4	Tympanic membrane adherent to the promontory

▌ Investigations

Pure tone audiometry, including air conduction and appropriately masked bone conduction, is an essential part of the assessment and should be performed within 3 months of surgery.

Imaging of the temporal bone is not usually required for a simple perforation. If there is cholesteatoma and a concurrent mastoidectomy procedure is planned, a high resolution fine-cut CT scan of the temporal bones is recommended to act as a 'road map' for surgery.

MYRINGOPLASTY

▌ Aims of surgery

The principal aims of surgery are to provide the patient with an intact tympanic membrane resulting in a safe and dry ear that hears as well as possible.

▌ Alternatives to surgery

In addition to discussing surgery, it is important to advise patients of the alternatives available to them. In the case of a central perforation, these include observation coupled with water precautions, particularly if there are few symptoms and the impact on lifestyle is minimal. A trial of a hearing aid is an option if hearing loss is the primary symptom.

Complications

- Scar (potential for poor cosmesis).
- Bleeding.
- Infection.
- Graft failure (personal audit will determine this risk – 10%–30%).
- Chorda tympani injury with taste disturbance (usually temporary).
- Ear numbness (particularly with a post-auricular incision).
- Hearing loss (dead ear <1%).
- Tinnitus (rare).
- Vertigo (rare).
- Facial nerve palsy (usually temporary and rare).

OPERATIVE PROCEDURE

Preoperatively, it is important to ensure the patient is adequately marked, has an up-to-date audiogram within 3 months and still has the perforation (Figure 14.1).

Figure 14.1. Tympanic membrane perforation.

Do not assume that the anaesthetist is familiar with the type of surgery planned. In particular, discuss the need for intraoperative hypotension to reduce bleeding and lack of paralysis to enable facial nerve monitoring.

Patients are placed supine, with their head on a head ring, rotated away from the operative ear.

A small amount of hair removal may be required. We recommend the use of a facial nerve monitor if it is used for all otological cases (other than insertion of a grommet). The entire theatre team becomes familiar with how to set it up and there is no ambiguity as to whether it is required for a particular procedure. It is also useful in the event of any unexpected pathology. Strapping patients to the table is helpful and allows them to be rotated during surgery, which can improve visualization of middle ear structures. A useful check list prior to scrubbing up is to consider five Ss:

- *Side* – correct side?
- *Spikes* – facial nerve monitor.
- *Straps* – is the patient secured to the table?
- *Scan* – has the scan been checked?
- *Shave* – is hair removal adequate?

▮ Procedure steps

Injection of local anaesthetic

The use of a local anaesthetic such as 2% with 1:80,000 adrenaline is used to aid vasoconstriction and postoperative analgesia. The procedure can be performed under local anaesthetic, but general anaesthesia is more common. The ear canal skin is infiltrated with local anaesthetic providing hydrodissection, thus making it easier to dissect and less likely to bleed. The site of any intended external incision is then infiltrated.

Remove margins of the perforation

With the perforation clearly in view a gently curved needle can be used to make a series of tiny perforations around it (Figure 14.2). It is helpful to start inferiorly and work superiorly to prevent bleeding from the edge obscuring the view. The small perforations are joined together and the inner ring of tissue can be gently pulled away using crocodile or cupped forceps leaving a freshened and slightly larger perforation.

Figure 14.2. Incision and freshening the edge of the perforation.

Incision

There are three standard approaches for performing otological procedures. The choice usually comes down to surgeon preference. Adequate exposure of the entire perforation is essential and will influence which approach is used. It may also be necessary to perform a limited canalplasty to remove any bone obscuring the view of the perforation, particularly if there is an anterior canal wall overhang obscuring an anterior perforation.

- *Permeatal* – If the external auditory canal (EAC) permits a view of the entire perforation and is wide enough to accommodate a large speculum, this approach can be used for both small and large perforations. It is helpful to use as wide a speculum as the EAC will allow. This can be secured with a clear plastic drape.
- *Postauricular* – A curved incision is made approximately 1 cm behind the postauricular crease through the skin and subcutaneous tissue onto the temporalis fascia in its upper half. A semicircular incision is made through the periosteum just posterior to the bony EAC. The skin of the posterior EAC is then elevated prior to making a re-entry incision into the EAC.

Tapes passed through the ear canal and out via the reentry incision can be used to retract the pinna and lateral meatal skin out of the field of view.

- *Preauricular (endaural)* – An incision is made just anterior to the anterior helix of the pinna and runs inferiorly between the helix and the tragus. It is continued into the roof of the EAC. A limb can be extended down the posterior wall of the EAC. The meatal skin lateral to this limb can then be elevated laterally over the bony margin of the ear canal. A two-prong retractor is then used to give exposure.

Tympanomeatal flap

Whatever approach is used, it is usually necessary to elevate a tympanomeatal flap,

Figure 14.3. Tympanomeatal flap.

except in cases of very small perforations, where a fat or fascial graft can be 'tucked' through the perforation. A posteriorly placed bucket handle incision is made, extending from the 12 o'clock position of the tympanic membrane (TM) (adjacent to the lateral process of the handle of malleus) to beyond the 6 o'clock position (Figure 14.3). Microscissors are required for the thicker meatal skin of the superior EAC. The flap is elevated using an elevator such as a Rosen ring until the annulus is reached. A fine elevator such as a Hugh's is used to elevate the annulus and enter the middle ear. By entering the middle ear postero-inferiorly, injury to the chorda tympani is minimized. Once the TM is reflected anteriorly along the handle of the malleus (Figure 14.1), it should be possible to see the medial surface of the anterior extent of the perforation. For a larger perforation, it is helpful to elevate the TM off the handle of malleus. An ophthalmic keratome knife is extremely useful for dividing the adherent fibres attaching the TM to the umbo.

Check the ossicular chain

Visually inspect the ossicles, in particular the incudostapedial joint (ISJ). Gently palpate the malleus handle and observe the movement of the malleus and incus (limited if there is attic fixation), confirm the integrity of the ISJ and mobility of the stapes footplate.

Graft harvest

The two commonest graft materials used are temporalis fascia and a composite cartilage perichondrium graft. Temporalis fascia is simply harvested via a post- or preauricular incision. To enable it to be easier to manipulate, it is scraped flat and left to dry. Cartilage can be harvested from the concha cymba, concha cavum or fossa triangularis if using a post-auricular incision, or from the tragus if performing a permeatal or end-aural approach. The composite perichondrium cartilage graft technique uses a single shield or island-shaped graft that remains attached to its perichondrium to reconstruct part or all of the tympanic membrane. Cartilage composite grafts have a very high success rate for repair of both small and large perforations, and are resilient to retraction without adversely affecting hearing outcomes (3).

Graft sizing

A helpful technique is to cut a paper template to accurately size the perforation or region of tympanic membrane that requires reconstruction. If using fascia, the graft will need to be bigger than the template. If using a composite island graft, the cartilage can be trimmed to the size of the perforation, while retaining a perichondrial apron to aid with graft placement.

Graft placement

The graft is placed beneath the tympanic membrane in an underlay fashion (Figure 14.4) and manipulated such that the entire TM defect is sealed (Figure 14.5). The graft should lie flat against the undersurface of the TM. If using a composite graft, the perichondrium lies laterally on the undersurface of the TM. Surface tension is usually adequate to keep the graft in place, but additional support can be obtained by placing small Gelfoam™ or Spongostan™ pieces in the middle ear. The tympanomeatal flap is then relocated in its original position.

Figure 14.4. Underlay composite cartilage 'island' graft.

Figure 14.5. Graft in position.

Ear packing

The surface of the tympanic membrane is gently covered to protect it and allow epithelium to grow over the graft. The dressing used is dependent on the preference of the surgeon. This can be done with a thin strip of clear silastic, small pieces of BIPP ribbon gauze or with gel foam blocks. The external auditory canal is then filled with further short strips of BIPP ribbon gauze (or similar) or a Pope wick in order to keep the meatal skin in place and prevent blunting of the angle between the TM and ear canal.

Closure

The wounds are closed in layers, preferably with an absorbable suture such as 4/0 Vicryl or Monocryl. A head bandage may or may not be required (4 hours is usually adequate).

POSTOPERATIVE REVIEW

Postoperatively it is good practice to document the facial nerve function and to confirm that there is still hearing in the operated ear by performing a Weber test. The majority of myringoplasty cases can be performed as day surgery, particularly if performed permeatally.

Advise the patient to keep the ear dry until after review. Postoperative follow-up is usually 2–4 weeks after surgery, at which time the dressings are removed from the ear.

KEY POINTS:

- Audiometry – Ensure the patient has an up-to-date, ear-specific, appropriately masked audiogram within 3 months prior to surgery.
- CT scan – A high-resolution temporal bone CT scan provides a useful 'roadmap' for mastoid surgery.
- Facial nerve monitor – Make it a routine part of your practice.
- Correct side.
- Optimal access and visualization. The local anaesthetic, hypotensive general anaesthetic, surgical approach and ability to manoeuvre the operating table combine to provide the best surgical conditions.

REFERENCES

1 Wullstein H. 1956. Theory and practice of tympanoplasty. *Laryngoscope* 66: 1976–93.
2 Sade J, Berco E. 1976. Atelectasis and secretory Otitis media. *American Journal of Otolaryngology* 85(Suppl. 25): 66–72.
3 Dornhoffer J. 2003. Cartilage tympanoplasty: Indications, techniques and outcomes in a 1000 patient series. *Laryngoscope* 113(11): 1844–56.

15 MASTOIDECTOMY

Neil Donnelly and Olivia Kenyon

Mastoidectomy is the surgical removal of all or part of the petromastoid portion of the temporal bone. The degree of removal depends on the condition being addressed.

Indications

- *For pathology* – Removal of disease within the mastoid air cells or from the middle ear, including acute mastoiditis, malignancy, mucosal chronic secretory otitis media (CSOM) and, most commonly, CSOM with cholesteatoma.
- *For access* – The mastoid component of the temporal bone acts as a conduit for a number of surgical procedures, including hearing implantation surgery (cochlear and middle ear), endolymphatic sac surgery, labyrinth surgery (posterior or superior semicircular canal occlusion and osseous labyrinthectomy) and translabyrinthine approaches to the internal auditory canal and cerebellopontine angle (vestibular schwannoma surgery).

CHOLESTEATOMA SURGERY

Cholesteatoma is keratinizing squamous epithelium (skin cells) within the middle ear space. They tend to gradually enlarge. The combination of enzyme production and pressure necrosis can result in the destruction of bony structures, including the ossicles and otic capsule.

ASSESSMENT

History

Cholesteatomas typically present with a painless discharging ear (often with an unpleasant odour) and an associated hearing loss. Less commonly, they can present with one of the more serious complications of CSOM with cholesteatoma, including meningitis, acute mastoiditis, facial nerve palsy and vertigo secondary to a lateral semicircular canal fistula. As with any otological procedure, the condition of the contralateral ear is an important consideration.

Examination

Document the origin of the cholesteatoma. Does it originate in the attic, from a marginal perforation or a pars tensa retraction pocket? Describe the status of the middle ear (dry or infected?) including the state of the ossicular chain. Document the state of the contralateral ear.

▌ Investigations

Pure tone audiometry, including air conduction and appropriately masked bone conduction, is an essential part of the assessment and should be performed within 3 months of surgery.

An axial high-resolution fine-cut CT scan of the temporal bones with coronal reconstructions is an important component of management. This is not performed for diagnostic purposes, which is clinical, but serves as a 'roadmap' for planning surgery to determine:

● The extent of cholesteatoma (often unreliable).
● Whether the sigmoid sinus is dominant or situated anteriorly.
● The level of the middle fossa dura and whether this is dehiscent.
● The course of the facial nerve and whether this is dehiscent.
● Whether there is erosion of the otic capsule.
● The state of the ossicles.

A number of different mastoidectomy techniques can be employed in the treatment of cholesteatoma. These include:

● Combined approach tympanoplasty (CAT), also known as a canal wall up mastoidectomy (Figure 15.1(a)).

(a)

(b)

(c)

Figure 15.1. (a) Combined approach tympanoplasty. (b) Attico antrostomy. (c) Modified radical mastoidectomy.

- Atticotomy or small cavity mastoidectomy, also known as front-to-back mastoidectomy (Figure 15.1(b)). This is increasingly combined with an endoscopic approach.
- Modified radical mastoidectomy also known as a canal wall down mastoidectomy (Figure 15.1(c)).

A good otologist should be trained in all three techniques so that the procedure performed can be tailored to the specific disease and requirements of the patient.

AIMS OF SURGERY

The principal aims of surgery are to provide the patient with a safe, dry ear that hears to the best of its ability and to eradicate the risks associated with untreated cholesteatoma.

ALTERNATIVES TO SURGERY

When discussing surgery, it is important to advise patients of the alternatives available to them. In the case of cholesteatoma, surgery is the only means of eradicating the disease and the associated complications. Observation is an option in selected cases, in particular, in patients who are symptom-free, too unfit for surgery or who decline surgery.

Cholesteatoma in an only hearing ear is not an absolute contraindication to surgery, but it is advisable that any procedure be undertaken by an experienced otologist.

Complications

The risks of surgery include:

- Scar (potential for poor cosmesis).
- Bleeding.
- Infection.
- Residual or recurrent disease (up to 25% with CAT, hence the need for second-look surgery).
- Facial nerve injury (<1%).
- Chorda tympani injury with taste disturbance (usually temporary even if the chorda is divided).
- Ear numbness (particularly with postauricular incision).
- Hearing loss (risk of dead ear up to 1%).
- Tinnitus (rare).
- Vertigo (rare).

OPERATION

Preoperatively, it is important to ensure the patient is adequately marked and has an up-to-date audiogram. Review the CT scan and determine whether any complicating factors are anticipated.

Check the availability of any specialist equipment with the scrub team. This may include an adequate selection of the preferred ossicular replacement prostheses, the availability of a KTP laser with appropriately trained operator or a range of otoendoscopes.

Ensure that the anaesthetist is aware of the need for intra-operative facial nerve monitoring and relative hypotension to reduce bleeding. A reinforced endotracheal tube is preferred to a laryngeal mask.

The patient is placed supine, with their head on a head ring, rotated away from the operative ear. A small amount of periauricular hair removal may be required. Most otologists regard the use of a facial nerve monitor for cholesteatoma surgery as mandatory if the hospital is in possession of the device. Strapping patients to the table is extremely helpful and allows them to be rotated during surgery to improve visualization of difficult areas. Many surgeons mark the planned postaural incision and mastoid process (Figure 15.2(a)). A useful checklist prior to scrubbing up is to consider five Ss:

- *Side* – is the side correct?
- *Spikes* – facial nerve monitor.
- *Straps* – is the patient secured to the table?
- *Scan* – has the CT scan been checked?
- *Shave* – is hair removal adequate?

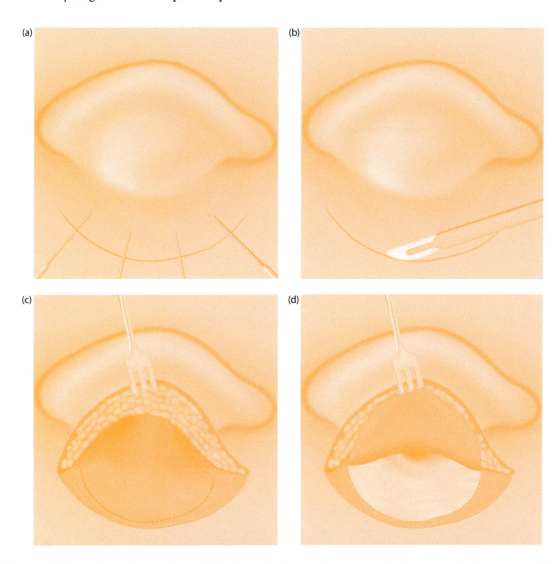

Figure 15.2. (a) Local anaesthetic infiltration. (b) Postaural incision. (c) Cutaneous incision elevated in superficial temporal plane. (d) Anteriorly based periosteal flap.

Combined Approach Tympanoplasty

Procedure steps

1 *Injection of local anaesthetic* – The use of a local anaesthetic such as 2% xylocaine with 1:80,000 adrenaline is used to infiltrate the canal skin and the region of the postauricular incision (Figures 15.2(a) and (b)).

2 *Incision (postauricular)* – A curved incision is made 1–2 cm behind the postauricular crease through skin and subcutaneous tissue onto loose aorta tissue lateral to temporalis fascia in its upper half (Figure 15.2(c)). An incision is made through the periosteum of the mastoid and an anteriorly based subperiosteal flap raised (Figure 15.2(d)) using a periosteal elevator. The skin of the posterior EAC is then elevated prior to making a reentry incision into the EAC. Tapes passed through the ear canal and out via the reentry incision are used to keep the pinna and lateral meatal skin retracted.

This approach provides excellent exposure of the cortical bone of the mastoid and the root of the zygomatic process.

3 *Tympanomeatal flap and disease isolation* – The goal is to isolate the middle ear component of the cholesteatoma, while preserving the healthy remnant of the tympanic membrane. As with a myringoplasty, a posteriorly placed bucket handle incision is made, extending from the 12 o'clock position of the TM (adjacent to the lateral process of the handle of malleus) to beyond the 6 o'clock position. The superior aspect of the tympanomeatal flap incision is taken right up to the margin of cholesteatoma. Microscissors are used to cut around the neck of the cholesteatoma. It may be necessary to divide the chorda tympani cleanly if it is involved in the disease. The resulting flap of posterior canal skin and tympanic membrane remnant is elevated and reflected anteroinferiorly. At the same time, the TM may be elevated off the handle of malleus. An ophthalmic keratome knife is useful for dividing the adherent fibres attaching the TM to the umbo ("Llyod's ligament").

4 *Check the ossicular chain* – Visually inspect the ossicles and their relationship with the cholesteatoma. If the ossicular chain is intact, a decision regarding whether it will be possible to clear disease adequately without disrupting it must be made. With a more extensive cholesteatoma involving the mesotympanum, it may be necessary to remove disease in order to get a view of the incus and or stapes. In these cases, there is often erosion of the long process of the incus. If the incudostapedial joint is intact, it is divided with a joint knife and the incus carefully removed without damaging the stapes superstructure. The neck of the malleus is then divided with malleus nippers and the head of the malleus removed; the handle of malleus can either be removed or left in situ. Removal of the handle of malleus can make reconstruction simpler and reduce recurrent cholesteatoma.

5 *Cortical mastoidectomy* – Using a 5 or 6 mm cutting burr, the cortical bone is removed to make a cavity, the superior margin of which is the tegmen tympani, posterior margin the sigmoid sinus and anterior margin the bony wall of the external auditory canal. As bone is removed, air cells will come into view depending on the degree of sclerosis of the mastoid. It is important to find the tegmen and sigmoid sinus and then skeletonize them (leave a thin layer of bone) with a diamond burr. This ensures that optimal access is achieved and that the surgeon does not become lost down a deep dark hole. The bone of the posterior canal is thinned while looking into the cavity and down the EAC. With progressive bone removal, the mastoid antrum is encountered. With the mastoid antrum open, the bony bulge of the lateral semicircular canal comes into view, as does the lateral process of the incus. Extreme caution is required as drilling on an intact ossicular chain may result in a sensorineural hearing loss. Anterosuperiorly, the dissection continues forward with a smaller cutting burr

into the root of the zygomatic process between the tegmen and bone of the superior EAC to provide access to the attic. The dissection is continued anteriorly until the anterior attic is accessible; this can otherwise be a common site for residual disease. Throughout the procedure, cholesteatoma and granulations may require piecemeal removal in order to maintain visualization. The final cavity should be smooth and disease-free.

6 *Posterior tympanotomy* – This refers to the removal of the triangle of bone between the facial nerve, chorda tympani and fossa incudis and is best performed with a small diamond burr. The first step is to find the mastoid segment of the facial nerve while drilling parallel to it with copious irrigation. Once located, it is possible to remove the bone lateral to the nerve in order to encounter the intra-osseous chorda. By removing the bone between the facial nerve and chorda tympani, the facial recess is opened, providing a view of the stapes (if present) and sinus tympani. In addition to the anterior attic, the sinus tympani is a frequent site for residual cholesteatoma; a good posterior tympanotomy provides optimal visualization of this tricky area which can be supplemented with angled otoscopes.

7 *Tympanic membrane reconstruction* – A composite cartilage graft (cartilage and perichondrium) is an excellent material for this and has a high resilience to retraction without adversely affecting hearing outcomes (1). Cartilage is harvested from the concha cymba or concha cavum via the postauricular incision. The posterior bony annulus and attic are smoothed off. A tape passed through the canal and brought out through the mastoid cavity can be used to remove residual squames from the bony margin. A paper template is prepared to size the attic and tympanic membrane reconstruction is required.

This is done prior to harvesting the cartilage to ensure a large enough piece of cartilage is taken. Once harvested, the cartilage is shaped to the template (taking care to place the lateral aspect of the template on the cartilage) leaving a peripheral apron of perichondrium surrounding the cartilage. The cartilage is scored down to perichondrium, twice horizontally and twice vertically. The result is nine separate pieces, resembling a chessboard, that are attached to the perichondrium. This technique removes the natural convexity of conchal cartilage and makes the graft easier to manipulate in the ear. The graft is placed in the middle ear in an underlay fashion with the perichondrium laterally. The perichondrium is placed over the bony meatal wall, lateral to the bony annulus, but medial to the annular ligament and tympanomeatal flap, to anchor the graft and prevent medialization. The cartilage should extend snugly to the bony annulus or overlap if there is concern about recurrence.

8 *Ossiculoplasty* – A partial or total ossicular replacement prosthesis (typically titanium or hydroxyapatite) is positioned to bridge the ossicular gap between the tympanic membrane and stapes head or footplate respectively. The head of the prosthesis lies against the undersurface of the cartilage checkerboard.

9 *Ear packing* – The surface of the reconstructed tympanic membrane is gently covered with small pieces of BIPP ribbon gauze, or alternative ear pack such as Gelfoam®. The ossiculopasty is inspected via the posterior tympanotomy to ensure that this remains in an optimal position prior to filling the external auditory canal with additional short strips of BIPP ribbon gauze.

10 *Closure* – The postauricular wound is closed in layers with absorbable sutures, packing head bandage with mastoid dressing is placed if required.

Postoperatively, the facial nerve function is documented. A postoperative lower motor neurone palsy is extremely worrying and the operating surgeon must be informed. While the palsy may be due to the local anesthetic, if the nerve fails to recover, surgical exploration by the operating surgeon and a second senior otologist is required. Facial nerve re-anastamosis may be attempted.

A Weber test or scratch test is also performed to confirm that there is still hearing in the operated ear. While the majority of mastoidectomy cases require an overnight stay, an increasing number are being performed as day-case procedures.

Patients are is advised to keep their ear dry until after review. Postoperative follow-up is usually 2 weeks after surgery, at which time the dressings are removed. Postoperative antibiotics are not usually necessary.

REFERENCE

1 Dornhoffer J. 2003. Cartilage tympanoplasty: indications, techniques and outcomes in a 1,000 patient series. *Laryngoscope* 113(11): 1844–56.

16 STAPEDECTOMY

Neil Donnelly and Olivia Kenyon

Stapedectomy literally means the surgical removal of the stapes bone. The term has come to refer to the operation in which the stapes superstructure is replaced by an artificial piston attached to the incus (typically) and placed through a fenestration in the stapes footplate (stapedotomy). This procedure is used to correct the conductive hearing loss that arises as a result of otosclerosis (Figure 16.1).

Figure 16.1. Stapedectomy typically involves removal of the stapes crura, fenestration of the footplate and the insertion of an artificial piston.

Otosclerosis affects the bone of the otic capsule, leading to new bone formation around the edge of the oval window and stapes footplate. Eventually, the stapes becomes fixed, resulting in reduced transmission of sound to the cochlea and significant conductive hearing loss.

ASSESSMENT

▌ History

The typical presenting symptom of otosclerosis is hearing loss. Less often there may be associated tinnitus or vertigo. It is commonly (70%) a bilateral condition in patients with a family history of hearing loss. Otosclerosis genes are transmitted in an autosomal dominant manner. However, due to variable penetrance and expression, it does not affect every generation.

Examination

Tuning fork tests are useful to confirm clinically a conductive hearing loss. It is necessary to document the state of both ears and exclude other causes of conductive hearing loss (e.g. otitis media with effusion or a retraction pocket with ossicular erosion). In active disease, hypervascularity of the promontory may be seen as a pinkish blush through the tympanic membrane. This is known as Schwartze's sign.

Investigations

Pure tone audiometry including air conduction and appropriately masked bone conduction, is an essential part of the assessment. In early disease, a predominantly lowfrequency conductive hearing loss is found. With increased fixation of the stapes, higher frequencies become affected. There may be a mixed conductive and sensorineural loss if there is additional cochlear otosclerosis. Characteristically, a Carhart's notch is seen, where a dip in the bone conduction occurs maximally at 2 kHz. This is due to the loss of the middle ear component of sound conduction at this natural frequency of resonance of the ossicular chain.

Tympanometry demonstrates a normal type A tympanogram, confirming normal middle ear compliance. Stapedial reflexes are typically absent on the affected side.

Speech audiometry can be a useful investigation, particularly in the presence of a mixed hearing loss. Maximum speech discrimination scores (SDS) of less than 70% may be associated with a poorer perceived benefit from surgery.

AIMS OF SURGERY

The principal aims of stapedectomy are to provide the patient with an ear that hears to the best of its ability. The probability of improving the hearing to within 10 dB of the bone conduction is >90%.

ALTERNATIVES TO SURGERY

In addition to discussing surgery, it is important to advise patients of the alternatives available to them. Many patients will elect for observation once the diagnosis has been made.

A trial of a hearing aid is a riskfree and effective option that should be encouraged prior to electing for surgery. Another alternative is a bone conduction device such as BAHA.

Complications

The risks of surgery include:

- Bleeding.
- Infection.
- Chorda tympani injury with taste disturbance.
- Dead ear or hearing loss (approximately 1%).
- Failure to close the air–bone gap within 10 dB (approximately 5%).
- Late failure.
- Tinnitus.
- Vertigo.
- Facial nerve injury (rare).

OPERATION

The side to be operated on should be clearly marked and the risks of the procedure explained. The ear must be dry, with no active infection. A recent (within 3 months) audiogram should also be present.

Check the availability of any specialist equipment with the scrub team. This includes an adequate selection of the preferred stapedectomy prosthesis and, depending on the technique used, a KTP laser with an appropriately trained operator.

As with other otological procedures, ensure the anaesthetist is aware of the need for intra-operative facial nerve monitoring and relative hypotension to reduce bleeding.

Patients are placed supine, with their head on a head ring, rotated away from the operative ear. A small sandbag is placed beneath the shoulders to extend the neck as this makes it easier to access the posterosuperior region of the tympanic membrane. As with other otological cases, facial nerve monitoring and strapping the patient to the table can be useful adjuncts.

▮ Stapedectomy

Procedure steps

1 *Injection of local anaesthetic* – Local anaesthetic (e.g. 2% xylocaine with 1:80 000 adrenaline) is used to infiltrate the canal skin in order to thicken the tympanomeatal flap and reduce bleeding. It is common practice in many clinics to perform the entire procedure under local anaesthesia, with a periauriclar block.

2 *Incision* – Typically a permeatal or endaural approach is used.

3 *Tympanomeatal flap* – A posterior bucket handle incision is made, extending from the 12 o'clock position of the TM to the 6 o'clock position. The meatal incision should not be too close to the annulus as it is often necessary to remove some of the bony annulus. The tympanomeatal flap is raised, hinged along the malleus and out of the way, providing access to the posterior contents of the mesotymanum and allowing the necessary view of the long process of incus, incudostapedial joint, stapedius tendon and stapes footplate. If access is limited, a House curette is used to remove the bone posterior and superior to the stapes until the desired view is achieved (Figure 16.2(a)).

4 *Check of the ossicular chain* – Palpate the ossicular chain with a needle. Confirm that the stapes footplate is fixed and that the malleus and incus are mobile.

5 *Division of the incudostapedial joint (ISJ)* – The ISJ is divided with a joint knife or fine right-angled hook. The joint can be clearly identified by gently elevating the incus. Division of the joint should be in line with, and away from, the stapedius tendon.

6 *Division of the stapedius tendon* – The stapedius tendon is divided with a laser, sharp sickle knife or microscissors.

7 *Removal of stapes superstructure* – The posterior crus of the stapes is divided with a laser or skeeter drill. The anterior crus is divided by down-fracturing towards the promontory (Figure 16.2(b)).

8 *Fenestration* – A small fenestration (stapedotomy) is made in the stapes footplate using a skeeter drill, laser or hand-held trephine. The fenestration typically has a diameter of 0.8 or 0.7 mm to accommodate a 0.6 mm prosthesis (Figure 16.2(c)).

9 *Prosthesis* – A stapedectomy prosthesis is placed within the fenestration and secured around the long process of the incus (Figure 16.2(d)). Small pieces of fat, harvested from the ear lobule, are placed around the prosthesis to prevent leakage of perilymph. A vein graft may be placed over the fenestration to perform the same task.

10 *Ear packing* – The tympanomeatal flap is replaced and the ear lightly packed with small pieces of BIPP ribbon gauze/sponge.

Figure 16.2. Steps involved when performing a stapedectomy. (a) Elevated tympanomeatal flap. (b) Divided stapedius tendon and stapes crura. (c) Fenestrated footplate. (d) Artificial stapes piston in place.

POSTOPERATIVE REVIEW

The facial nerve function is documented and a Weber test is performed to confirm that there is still hearing in the operated ear. The eyes are examined and any nystagmus noted. While some stapedectomy cases require an overnight stay, increasing numbers are being performed as day-case procedures.

Patients are given advice to keep their ear dry until after review, and to avoid straining. Postoperative follow-up is usually 2 weeks after surgery, at which time the dressings are removed.

17 BONE-ANCHORED HEARING AID

James Tysome

A bone-anchored hearing aid (BAHA) provides hearing rehabilitation through bone conduction. The BAHA consists of a titanium implant, abutment and a sound processor. The implant is placed surgically into the skull behind the ear and forms a solid attachment to bone through osseo-integration. The abutment traverses the subcutaneous tissues and skin to allow attachment of the sound processor. This facilitates sound conduction through vibrations, which are transmitted via the abutment and implant complex and through the skull to reach the cochlea. BAHA offers superior sound quality to a conventional bone conductor hearing aid.

Indications

- Patients unable to wear a conventional hearing aid due to otitis externa, chronically discharging ears despite middle ear surgery, allergy to hearing aid moulds or congenital malformation of the middle or external ear, including canal and pinna atresia.
- Unilateral complete sensorineural hearing loss. Placed behind the deaf ear, the BAHA facilitates the conduction of sound through the skull to the good ear. This prevents the head shadow effect from the deaf side, although in general does not improve directionality.

PREOPERATIVE REVIEW

Ensure that patients have completed their audiological assessment for BAHA, which includes a trial of a bone conductor worn on a headband. Mark the side on which the BAHA is to be placed.

OPERATIVE PROCEDURE

The implants have become wider over recent years, allowing longer abutments up to 14 mm to be safely used. This has resulted in the use of a tissue preservation technique without the need for a skin flap or thinning of subcutaneous tissues. This has resulted in shorter operative time and retention of the normal hair that grows back around the abutment, with a vast decrease in infections that cause most long-term problems with BAHAs.

The surgery is now usually performed under local anaesthetic. The patient is positioned supine with the head facing 45° away from the surgeon. Shave the postauricular area, prepare the skin and drape (Figure 17.1(a)).

Mark the position of the implant 55 mm from the external auditory meatus in the direction shown (Figure 17.1(b)). Use the dummy sound processor

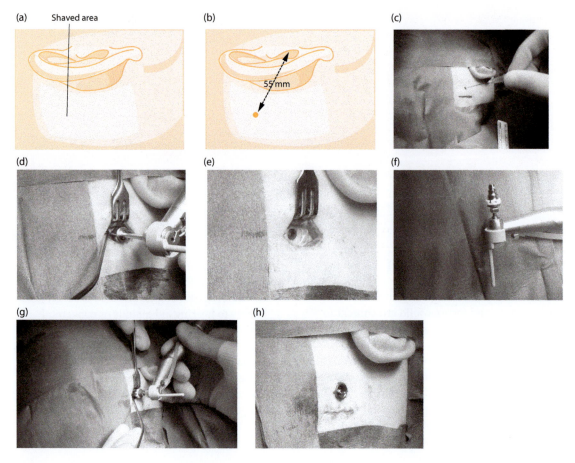

Figure 17.1. (a) Postauricular shave. (b) Marking implant position and incision. (c) Linear skin incision. (d) Drilling. (e) Countersunk hole ready for implant. (f) Implant and abutment mounted on drill for one-stage insertion. (g) Placing implant and abutment together. (h) Implant complete.

in order to ensure that the eventual position of the processor will not impinge on the ear and the arm of glasses if worn. Measure the skin depth at the mark using a needle. This allows calculation of the appropriate abutment length to traverse the skin. Methylene blue can also be used to mark the implant site on the periosteum. A 2 cm linear incision is marked 1 cm from the proposed implant position (Figure 17.1(c)).

Local anaesthesia (2% xylocaine, 1:80,000 adrenaline) is instilled and an incision made down to the periosteum. Tissues are elevated until the blue implant site mark is seen on the periosteum.

A cruciate incision is made in the periosteum and the corners elevated to access the bone. Drill the hole for the implant, using the hand-held drill with sufficient irrigation. Drill a 3 mm guide perpendicular to the skull. Palpate the base of the hole carefully to ensure that dura is not exposed. If bone remains, deepen the hole to a depth of 4 mm. A countersink is then used to widen the hole (Figure 17.1(d), (e)).

One-stage implants are used in the majority of cases, consisting of the implant screw and abutment as one unit (Figure 17.1(f)). Mount the implant onto the drill using a no-touch technique.

The implant is a self-tapping screw. It is essential that this is placed perpendicular to the skull. (Figure 17.1(g)). Punch a hole in the overlying skin with a 4 mm dermatological punch and make radial incisions in order to enable the abutment to pass through the skin. The incision is closed (Figure 17.1(h)) and a non-adherent dressing applied and secured in place with a healing cap attached firmly to the abutment.

A two-stage technique may be used in children, particularly where a 3 mm implant is used where the 3 mm guide drill encounters dura. In this situation, the implant alone is inserted along with a cover screw. After osseointegration has taken place, around 3 months later, a hole can be punched through the skin and the abutment screwed onto the implant.

POSTOPERATIVE REVIEW AND FOLLOW-UP

Following observation according to the day surgery protocol, the patient can be discharged with analgesia. Initial follow-up is at 1 week to remove the healing cap and dressings. The patient is taught to care for their implant, which requires daily cleaning with a soft toothbrush. The hearing aid is fitted and programmed soon after.

Complications

- Infection.
- Bleeding or haematoma.
- Failure of implant.
- Cerebrospinal fluid leak.

18 PANENDOSCOPY

Ram Moorthy

Panendoscopy refers to the formal assessment of the upper aerodigestive tract using rigid endoscopes. The term encompasses a number of distinct procedures:

- Examination of the postnasal space (PNS).
- Pharyngoscopy.
- Laryngoscopy.
- Rigid oesophagoscopy.

On occasion, a rigid bronchoscopy may be required to complete a formal assessment of the upper aerodigestive tract.

PREOPERATIVE REVIEW

All imaging must be reviewed. Patients at risk of cervical spine injury should undergo a cervical spine x-ray. Loose teeth or dental crowns require extra precautions to prevent damage. Mouth opening and neck movement are assessed in the awake patient as this will impact the ease of the procedure.

OPERATIVE PROCEDURE

The light source and carrier are checked to make certain they are functioning correctly. An appropriate range of endoscopes, Hopkins rods and a variety of biopsy forceps must be available.

The procedure is undertaken under general anaesthesia and the patient placed supine on the operating table. Either a pillow or head ring and shoulder roll are used to allow the neck to be slightly flexed and the head extended to achieve the 'sniffing the morning air' position. The endotracheal or nasotracheal tube is secured, the former being secured on the left if the surgeon is right-hand dominant.

The eyes are taped closed and the head draped with the nose and mouth exposed. The body is draped leaving the neck exposed.

In all cases, the neck is inspected for scars and the neck palpated for masses and laryngeal crepitus. The oral cavity, tongue base and tonsils are also palpated. For all procedures, except examination of the PNS, an appropriate mouth guard is placed to protect the upper teeth. If the patient is edentulous a wet swab will suffice.

Biopsies, if required, are taken distal to proximal in order to ensure that bleeding does not obscure the surgeon's view.

19 DIRECT- AND MICROLARYNGOSCOPY

Ram Moorthy

Indications

- Laryngeal pathology (e.g. laryngeal carcinoma, laryngeal polyp, cord oedema).
- Investigation of a patient with an unknown primary.
- Investigation of a patient with dysphagia.
- Investigation of an unknown cause for airway symptoms.
- Removal of a foreign body.
- Investigation and management of a patient with a vocal cord palsy.
- Paediatric airway assessment.

OPERATIVE PROCEDURE

The patient is intubated with a microlaryngeal tube which is of a standard length but of smaller diameter to allow better visualization.

The mouth is held open with the non-dominant hand. The laryngoscope is gently inserted and the tongue followed until the oropharynx is reached, with any secretions suctioned.

The endotracheal tube acts as a guide and can be followed directly to the larynx. Inspect the lingual and laryngeal surfaces of the epiglottis and the remainder to the supraglottis including the arytenoids. Once the vocal cords including the anterior commissure, are visible, the laryngoscope handle can be attached and the suspension arm fixed to the handle to support the laryngoscope when microlaryngoscopy is required. An anterior commissure laryngoscope which has a narrower cross-sectional profile, may be required to allow assessment of the anterior commissure.

A 0° Hopkins rod is passed through the lumen of the laryngoscope. Careful assessment is made of the supraglottis, glottis and subglottis and appropriate photographs taken. In paediatric patients, a probe is used to assess mobility of the cords and the cricoarytenoid joints. Representative biopsies can be taken from any lesions.

The operating microscope can now be used if the following procedures are undertaken (Figure 19.1):

- A magnified view of the larynx is required to allow accurate excision of a lesion or vocal cord injection.
- Both hands are required to perform the procedure.
- Laser excision of a laryngeal lesion.

Suspension arm

Microscope

Laryngoscope

Figure 19.1. Microlaryngoscopy. A laryngoscope is passed and suspended by its handle. A microscope provides a binocular view of the larynx.

Complications

- Bleeding.
- Infection.
- Damage to teeth, gums, lips and tongue.
- Hoarse voice.
- Sore throat.
- Dysphagia.
- Airway compromise, which may necessitate tracheostomy.

POSTOPERATIVE REVIEW

- If the patient is difficult to intubate and there is a high likelihood that the airway will be unstable on extubation, a tracheostomy should be undertaken.
- If there is any concern that the airway may be compromised, then extubation is performed in theatre and assessment of the airway undertaken prior to transfer to recovery. If there is any concern, reintubation and tracheostomy may be required.

Patients are advised to rest their voice for at least 48 hours, or to talk normally, with no shouting and/or whispering.

20 PHARYNGOSCOPY

Sonia Kumar

Indications

- Mass or ulcer of the oropharynx and hypopharynx.
- Investigation of a patient with an unknown primary.
- Dysphagia.
- Identifying a synchronous tumour in a patient with known malignancy of the upper aero-digestive tract.
- Removal of a foreign body.
- Globus sensation, failing to respond to medical therapy or with features suggestive of malignancy on history, examination or imaging.

OPERATIVE PROCEDURE

The non-dominant hand is used to gently open the mouth and the pharyngoscope inserted (Figure 20.1). The tongue will guide the surgeon inferiorly towards the oropharynx. Suction is required at this point, as secretions will obscure the surgical field. The tongue base, valleculae, tonsils, posterior and lateral pharyngeal walls are carefully examined.

The pharyngoscope is passed behind the endo-tracheal or nasotracheal tube in order to visualize the posterior pharyngeal wall, pyriform fossae and post-cricoid region.

It is essential that the surgeon has a clear view at all times. Never attempt to force the pharyngoscope as this risks causing an oesophageal perforation (Figure 20.2). If this leads to mediastinitis, the mortality rate is 50%. At the cricopharyngeal bar, the lumen may come to a blind end and the temptation is to push the scope blindly. Wait patiently for the muscle to relax. Otherwise, the larynx may be gently lifted forward to allow identification of the lumen

of the cervical oesophagus. The tip of the scope is advanced gently into the upper oesophagus. A 0° Hopkins rod can be passed through the lumen to

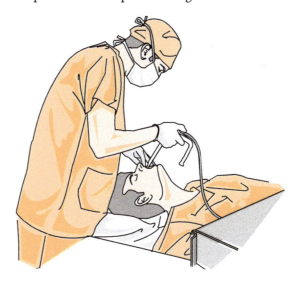

Figure 20.1. Insertion of the pharyngoscope.

Figure 20.2. At the cricopharyngeus, the scope is gently advanced in order to avoid tearing.

take photographs of any abnormality, prior to taking representative biopsies using an appropriate biopsy forceps (Figure 20.3). In patients with an unknown primary malignancy, biopsies of the tongue base and tonsils are usually taken if no obvious primary malignancy can be identified.

At the end of the procedure, ensure haemostasis and remove the teeth guard, checking for any

Figure 20.3. Suction is often required once the pharyngoscope is within the cervical oesophagus. Biopsy forceps are required if a biopsy is to be taken.

dental trauma which must be documented in the operation note.

POSTOPERATIVE REVIEW

If there is any concern of trauma to the upper oesophagus, a nasogastric tube should be passed under direct vision during the procedure and the patient kept nil by mouth. A contrast swallow allows visualization of a potential perforation. If the suspicion of perforation is low, the patient is observed closely for pain radiating to the back, pyrexia, tachycardia or tachypnoea. If these do not occur, the patient can commence sips of sterile water, gradually building up to free fluids and a soft diet prior to discharge home.

Complications

- Bleeding.
- Infection.
- Damage to teeth, gums, lips or tongue.
- Sore throat.
- Dysphagia.
- Hoarse voice.
- Damage to pharyngeal mucosa, including perforation.

21 RIGID OESOPHAGOSCOPY

Ram Moorthy

Rigid oesophagoscopy is performed in a similar manner to pharyngoscopy. Rigid oesophagoscopes are typically available 25 cm or 40 cm in length, which can reach the gastrooesophageal junction. It is important to ensure that suction and biopsy forceps of an appropriate length are available. A variety of appropriately shaped forceps are also available to help with foreign body removal.

Indications

- Similar to that for rigid pharyngoscopy.
- Removal of foreign body, especially star foreign bodies (bone) and batteries.
- To enable dilatation, with balloon or bougie, of stricture, stenosis or spasm.

OPERATIVE PROCEDURE

The procedure is performed under general anaesthesia. The airway is secured with an appropriately sized microlaryngoscopy tube.

The patient is positioned supine on the operating table with a head ring or equivalent, the lower cervical spine is flexed and the upper cervical spine is extended, as is the atlanto-occipital joint ('sniffing the morning air' position).

A mouth guard, or wet swab if edentulous, is placed to protect the teeth and gums. The procedure is similar to that for rigid pharyngoscopy. The tongue is followed back to the oropharynx and the oesophagoscope is passed behind the endotracheal or nasotracheal microlaryngoscopy tube. The oesophagoscope is manoeuvred into the post-cricoid region. The tip of the oesophagoscope is gently lifted to allow identification of the lumen of the oesophagus and the scope is gently advanced. Never force the

scope, especially if the lumen is not visible, which can traumatise the mucosa and potentially cause an oesophageal perforation.

If an abnormality is identified, use the etched marks on the oesophagoscope to estimate the distance from the incisors, and document this in the operation note. Representative biopsies are taken.

A soft food bolus obstruction can be pushed down and into the stomach.

Sharp foreign bodies must be removed with care to minimize trauma to the oesophageal mucosa. If possible the foreign body can be manoeuvred into the lumen of the oesophagoscope and the oesophagoscope removed.

Carefully assess the mucosa as the oesophagoscope is removed and, if there is any suspicion of a mucosal tear or perforation, a nasogastric tube is passed under direct vision prior to completing the procedure by removing the mouth guard or swab, checking the teeth and temporomandibular joint.

POSTOPERATIVE REVIEW

Where there is no suspicion of trauma to the oesophagus, patients can eat and drink normally. Otherwise, manage the patient as recommended for perforations after pharyngoscopy.

If a patient becomes pyrexic, tachycardic, tachypnoeic or has increasing retrosternal pain radiating through to their back or dysphagia, always assume they have suffered an oesophageal tear. These patients must be kept nil by mouth. They require IV antibiotics (as per local guidelines) and a nasogastric tube will need to be passed by the radiologists. Obtain an urgent chest x-ray to exclude a pneumomediastinum indicative of a tear, and inform a senior member of the team.

Complications

- As for rigid pharyngoscopy, risks include mucosal tear and perforation. Patients should be made aware of the risk of requiring a nasogastric tube and close monitoring in hospital for a few days if a perforation is suspected.

22 EXAMINATION OF POST NASAL SPACE

Sonia Kumar

Indications

- Mass or ulcer of the nasopharynx.
- Investigation of patients with an unknown primary.
- Persistent unilateral middle ear effusion in an adult.
- Unexplained epistaxis.

OPERATIVE PROCEDURE

This procedure is usually undertaken last if it is part of a panendoscopy, as any bleeding from the nasopharynx due to instrumentation can track into and obscure the view of the rest of the upper aerodigestive tract.

The patient is placed supine on the operating table and the head supported with a head ring. A decongestant or topical anaesthetic with adrenaline is applied to the nose, usually in the anaesthetic room.

A 0° Hopkins rod with an appropriate light source is passed into the nasal cavity, and the nasopharynx is carefully examined. The fossa of Rosenmüller in particular must be assessed, as this may harbour a malignancy. Biopsies are taken, if indicated, with straight Blakesley–Wilde or Tilley–Henckel forceps. Adrenaline-soaked neuropatties or diathermy can be applied if required for haemostasis.

Complications

- Bleeding/epistaxis.
- Infection.
- Otitis media with effusion secondary to inadvertent damage to the Eustachian tube orifice.

23 RIGID BRONCHOSCOPY

Sonia Kumar

Indications

- Removal of foreign body from the trachea or main bronchi.
- Assessment of a tracheal lesion.
- Assessment of subglottic or tracheal stenosis.

In many cases the proximal trachea can be assessed, as described in Chapter 24, with a laryngoscope and a 0° Hopkins rod.

OPERATIVE PROCEDURE

Bronchoscopes are available in a number of sizes. Selection of an appropriately sized bronchoscope is essential for paediatric patients. Before the patient is anaesthetized, ensure that the bronchoscope is assembled correctly and that the anaesthetic connectors are compatible (Figure 23.1). Confirm that the light source is working and that the camera has been attached. Appropriate optical forceps must be available if foreign body removal is required.

Safe bronchoscopy requires good teamwork and communication between the surgeon and the anaesthetist. When the patient is well oxygenated and the anaesthetist feels it is appropriate, the endotracheal tube or laryngeal mask is withdrawn and a mouth guard placed over the upper teeth. Using the anaesthetic laryngoscope, the larynx is visualized as the non-dominant hand supports the laryngoscope. The bronchoscope is held in the dominant hand and advanced until the larynx is reached. The bronchoscope may be rotated through 90° to facilitate passage through the glottic opening, which minimizes the risk damage to the vocal cord from the tip of the bronchoscope.

Once the bronchoscope is in the proximal trachea, the anaesthetic circuit is connected and the bronchoscope is advanced towards the carina. By gently turning the head to the left, the bronchoscope can be advanced into the right main bronchus, and vice versa. Secretions can be removed using narrow suction tubing, which can be advanced by an assistant or scrub nurse.

If a foreign body, especially an organic foreign body is visualized, it is vital that a small volume of 1:10,000 adrenaline is instilled via the suction tubing to reduce mucosal oedema and to allow vasoconstriction. This improves access and minimizes the risk of bleeding which can make removal of the foreign body very challenging. Appropriate optical forceps are then used to remove the foreign body. The bronchoscope is reinserted to ensure that there are no more foreign bodies and to assess for mucosal damage.

Figure 23.1. Diagram of a ventilating bronchoscope.

POSTOPERATIVE REVIEW

The patient is recovered in theatre to ensure that there are no breathing difficulties. If there has been mucosal damage, then a chest x-ray (CXR) is performed to exclude a pneumothorax.

Complications

These are similar to those for laryngoscopy. Others include:

- Damage to the vocal cords by the bronchoscope.
- Laryngospasm.
- Breathing difficulties due to airway oedema.
- Pneumothorax due to damage to the mucosa of the trachea or main bronchi.

24 SUBMANDIBULAR GLAND EXCISION

Ram Moorthy

This is a common surgical procedure performed by both ENT surgeons as well as oral and maxillofacial surgeons for benign and malignant disease.

The standard transcervical approach is described below. Nonstandard techniques include submental, retroauricular, transoral, endoscopic and robot-assisted surgery (1).

Indications

- Recurrent submandibular gland sialadenitis.
- Obstructive sialolithiasis.
- Benign tumours of the gland. If there is any suspicion of malignancy, then a Level I neck dissection is more appropriate than simple excision of the gland.
- Following open trauma to the gland, exploration and removal may be necessary to avoid salivary fistula formation.
- Drooling.

PREOPERATIVE REVIEW

Mark the operative side and check the function of the marginal mandibular, lingual and hypoglossal nerves.

Complications

- Bleeding.
- Infection.
- Marginal mandibular nerve damage: transient 5%–30% (1–3); permanent <1% (1).
- Lingual nerve damage – 2%–3% (1–3).
- Hypoglossal nerve damage.
- Salivary fistula.
- Scar.
- Recurrence (if surgery is for a tumour).
- Retained stone in stump of Wharton's duct.

OPERATIVE PROCEDURE

Once intubated and transferred to the operating table, position the patient supine on a head ring and shoulder roll with a slight head-up tilt. The head is turned to the contralateral side. The skin is appropriately prepared and draped to expose the corner of the mouth, and also the angle and lower border of the jaw to the superior border of the clavicle to the midline.

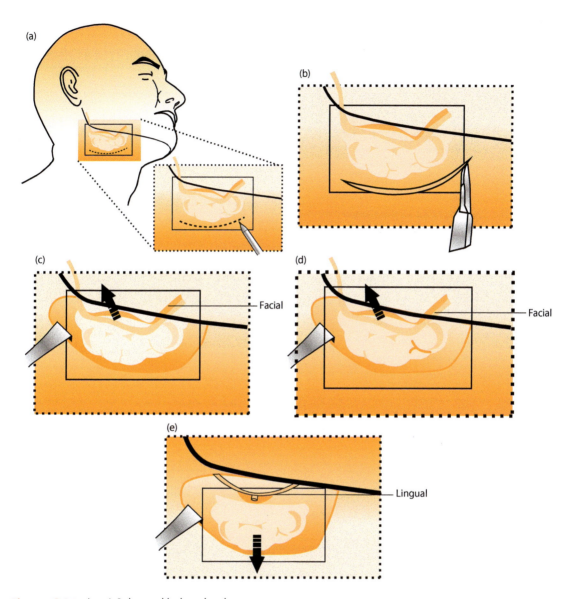

Figure 24.1. (a–e) Submandibular gland excision steps.

Mark the lower border of the mandible and the site of the skin incision, which lies two finger breadths (approx. 5 cm) below the lower border of the mandible, in order to avoid the marginal mandibular nerve (Figure 24.1(a)). The incision, ideally in a skin crease runs forward from the anterior edge of the sternocleidomastoid muscle and is approximately 5–7 cm in length (Figure 24.1(b)).

Make an incision through the skin, subcutaneous tissue and platysma. The marginal mandibular nerve can be damaged in the early stages of the procedure.

The nerve does not always have to be formally identified but knowledge of the relevant clinical anatomy is important as the nerve lies deep to the platysma but superficial to the gland and the facial vein. In some cases, especially for the management of malignant disease, identification of the nerve can be helpful to avoid iatrogenic injury, e.g. superficial to posterior facial vein as it crosses the mandible (4,5).

Stay close to the under-surface of the platysma and carefully observe for the nerve when elevating sub-platysmal flaps. The superficial layer of the deep cervical fascia is incised inferior to the lower border of the gland and elevated in an inferior to superior direction. The common facial vein is ligated and divided close to the inferior border of the gland and elevated superiorly away from the gland (Figure 24.1(c)). Ligation of the posterior facial vein near the inferior border of the gland and superior elevation with the investing fascia (Hayes–Martin manoeuvre) is an effective technique to avoid injury to the marginal mandibular nerve.

Once the gland is exposed, the facial artery is identified, ligated and divided. The gland is

retracted and dissected free of the underlying digastric muscle. The posterior border of the mylohyoid muscle is identified and the muscle is retracted anteriorly to allow dissection of the deep aspect of the gland.

The gland is retracted postero-inferiorly and, as dissection proceeds, Wharton's duct is exposed, which tents and exposes the lingual nerve and its ganglion (Figure 24.1(d)). The lingual nerve is dissected off the duct, paying careful attention to haemostasis, especially in the small plexus near the ganglion. The duct is followed and ligated as distally as possible to complete the excision. Occasionally, the facial artery will need to be ligated again as it courses over the mandible. The hypoglossal nerve is identified during dissection of the deep aspect of the gland (Figure 24.1(e)).

A drain may be inserted and the wound is closed in layers.

POSTOPERATIVE REVIEW

Examine the patient for nerve injury and haematoma. The drain can usually be removed in the morning and the patient discharged home with routine wound care advice.

Non-absorbable skin sutures are removed after seven days.

REFERENCES

1 Beahm DD et al. 2009. Surgical approaches to the submandibular gland. A review of literature. *Int J Surg* 7(6): 503–9.
2 Preuss SF, Klussmann JP, Wittekindt C, Drebber U, Beutner D, Guntinas-Lichius O. 2007. Sub-mandibular gland excision: 15 years of experience. *J Oral Maxillofac Surg* 65(5): 953–7.
3 Chua DY, Ko C, Lu KS. 2010. Submandibular mass excision in an Asian population: A 10-year review. *Ann Acad Med Singapore* 39(1): 33–7.
4 Ichimura K, Nibu K, Tanaka T. 1997. Nerve paralysis after surgery in the submandibular triangle: review of University of Tokyo Hospital experience. *Head Neck* 19(1): 48–53.
5 Riffat F, Buchanan MA, Mahrous AK, Fish BM, Jani P 2012. Oncological safety of the Hayes-Martin manoeuvre in neck dissections for node-positive oropharyngeal squamous cell carcinoma. *J Laryngol Otol* 126(10): 1045–8.

25 HEMI- AND TOTAL THYROIDECTOMY

Ram Moorthy

Indications

- Thyroid nodule or goitre.
  - Suspicious (usually hemi-thyroidectomy) or confirmed (usually total thyroidectomy) malignancy.
  - Compressive symptoms.
  - (Cosmesis).
- Thyrotoxicosis — a total thyroidectomy is usually undertaken.

Complications

- Bleeding.
- Infection.
- Scar.
- Hoarseness due to recurrent laryngeal nerve injury.
- Loss of the upper vocal range due to damage to the superior laryngeal nerve, which is especially important in singers.
- Breathing difficulties and, rarely, tracheostomy if bilateral vocal cord palsy after total thyroidectomy.
- Hypocalcaemia.
- Risk of requiring thyroid replacement following hemi-thyroidectomy alone.

PREOPERATIVE REVIEW

It is essential that all patients undergo a vocal cord check preoperatively to assess cord movement.

Review thyroid function tests and fine needle aspiration cytology (FNAC) results. Thyrotoxic patients are managed jointly with the endocrinologists in order to render them euthyroid to minimize the risk of an intraoperative thyroid storm.

Ensure the correct side is marked in a hemi-thyroidectomy.

OPERATIVE PROCEDURE

The patient is placed supine on the operating table with a shoulder roll and head ring. The skin is prepared and draped.

A nerve monitor may be used to monitor the integrity of the recurrent laryngeal nerve.

Monitoring may either be intermittent or continuous. The electrodes are typically attached or integrated into the endotracheal tube.

Surgery can be performed with standard instruments or with a variety of electrosurgical

Skin

Platysma muscle

Strap muscles

Sternocleidomastoid muscle

Thyroid gland

Internal jugular vein

Common carotid artery

Trachea

Recurrent laryngeal nerve

Oesophagus

Figure 25.1. Axial section through the neck at the level of the thyroid isthmus.

techniques or with the surgical robot now available.

A horizontal skin crease collar incision is made approximately 1–2 finger breadths (2.5–5 cm) above the sternal notch. Marking the incision prior to anaesthesia helps identify an appropriate skin crease.

The incision passes through skin, subcutaneous tissue and platysma (Figure 25.1). Sub-platysmal flaps are elevated as far as the superior thyroid notch superiorly and the supra-sternal notch inferiorly. The anterior jugular veins lie within the sub-platysmal plane and may require ligation and division. An appropriate retractor or sutures are used to retract the flaps out of the operative field.

The investing layer of deep fascia is incised and the strap muscles (sternothyroid and sternohyoid) lying in the midline will come into view. The strap muscles are separated in the midline. Sternothyroid may occasionally need to be divided for large goitres. This is performed as high as possible to preserve innervation from ansa hypoglossi.

The strap muscles are retracted laterally and the underlying gland dissected free, using a combination of sharp and blunt dissection.

The gland is freed in the para-carotid tunnel and the straps and carotid retracted laterally.

The superior pole is dissected from an inferior to superior direction. The superior vascular pedicle is isolated, ligated and divided close to the gland to minimize damage to the superior laryngeal nerve. This allows the superior pole to be freed from its fascial attachments.

The thyroid gland is retracted medially, which also rotates the larynx, exposing the tracheo-oesophageal groove. The middle thyroid vein is identified and divided. The recurrent laryngeal nerve (RLN) lies in the tracheo-oesophageal groove and has a variable course, but always enters the larynx at the cricothyroid joint. Safe identification of the RLN can be made in several ways including:

- The RLN runs within Beahrs' triangle, which is formed by the common carotid, inferior thyroid artery, and the recurrent laryngeal nerve. The RLN runs within Lore's triangle which is formed by the trachea, the carotid sheath and the under-surface of the inferior lobe of the thyroid.
- The RLN is related to the inferior thyroid artery, which is identified laterally at the external carotid and followed medially. The nerve is

usually deeper than the artery, but can be superficial or between its branches.

- Identify the RLN superiorly just before it enters the larynx caudal to the inferior pharyngeal constrictor.

Once the nerve has been identified, it is followed until it enters the larynx and the thyroid is carefully dissected free. It is vital that the parathyroid glands are identified and dissected free from the thyroid with their blood supply. Divide the inferior thyroid artery close to the thyroid gland to help achieve this.

The thyroid gland remains attached to the trachea by Berry's ligament, a dense fascial condensation. This is usually vascular and the gland is freed to the midline using bipolar and sharp dissection.

If a hemi-thyroidectomy is being performed, the isthmus is divided and over-sewn or transfixed, if required. If a total thyroidectomy is being performed, then the other lobe is excised in a similar fashion.

Haemostasis is achieved with the careful use of bipolar and great care taken around the nerve. A drain is optional.

The strap muscles are closed in the midline using an absorbable suture, with a gap left inferiorly to allow blood to escape from around the trachea and to minimize the risk of airway obstruction from a haematoma.

The wound is closed in layers.

POSTOPERATIVE REVIEW

A patient undergoing a total thyroidectomy or with a known vocal cord palsy is extubated in theatre and the patient's airway assessed prior to transfer to recovery.

Voice and cough should be assessed postoperatively. A bovine cough or weak and breathy voice indicates an RLN injury which should be confirmed by nasoendoscopy. Clip removers or scissors must always be at the patient's bedside to enable immediate evacuation of a haematoma should this occur with compromise of the airway.

If a completion hemi-thyroidectomy or total thyroidectomy has been undertaken, postoperative calcium levels may be checked after 4–6 hours and again the following morning. If the calcium

level is low, then the local protocol is followed in conjunction with the endocrinology team. Calcium may be replaced orally or, if very low, intravenously, with the addition of 1-α calcidol as required. The patient is also commenced on thyroid replacement with either levothyroxine (T) or, where radioactive iodine is to be administered within the following six weeks, liothyronine (T).

If a drain has been inserted, it is left in place overnight and removed when less than 20 mL has drained in a 24-hour period. The patient is discharged home once the drain has been removed and, if applicable, when the calcium is normal.

Vocal cord movement is assessed at outpatient follow-up.

26 SUPERFICIAL PAROTIDECTOMY

Ram Moorthy

The plane of the facial nerve divides the parotid gland anatomically into superficial and deep lobes, although they are functionally the same gland. The majority of parotid tumours occur in the superficial lobe. Superficial parotidectomy is excision of the parotid gland superficial to the facial nerve.

Indications

- Benign or malignant tumour of the parotid gland (most common).
- Chronic sialadenitis (rare).
- Sialolithiasis (rare).

Complications

- Facial weakness.
- Numbness of the ear lobe secondary to damage to the greater auricular nerve. This is to be expected in the majority of patients.
- Frey's syndrome. The cut parasympathetic nerve fibres reinnervate the sympathetic channels to supply the sweat glands in the cheek. Gustatory sweating occurs, which is sweating of the face on the side of surgery in anticipation of eating.
- Recurrence of tumour.
- Scar.
- Salivary fistula.
- Bleeding.
- Infection.

PREOPERATIVE REVIEW

Always check and document facial nerve function preoperatively (Figure 26.1). Review imaging, FNAC results and ensure that any preoperative blood test results are available.

OPERATIVE PROCEDURE

Once the patient has been intubated and transferred to the operating table, a head ring is placed under the head, a sandbag under the shoulder, and the head turned to the opposite side.

Facial nerve monitoring is used by most surgeons. Be familiar with the facial nerve monitor used in the unit, including correct placement of electrodes, connection to the monitor and checking correct function.

A cotton wool ball may be placed in the external auditory canal (EAC), The patient is prepared with aqueous iodine or chlorhexidine and draped

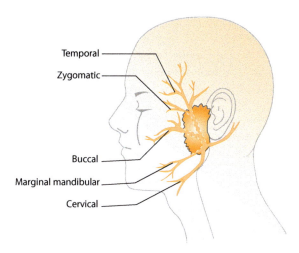

Temporal
Zygomatic

Buccal
Marginal mandibular
Cervical

Figure 26.1. External branches of the facial nerve.

to ensure that the majority of the face is exposed, especially the ipsilateral eye and corner of the mouth.

The most common incision used in the 'lazy-S' incision (Figure 26.2), although a face lift incision is becoming more popular. Infiltration with adrenaline alone, or local anaesthetic and adrenaline, may be used to provide some haemostasis.

Lazy-S incision

Figure 26.2. Incision landmarks for a parotidectomy.

Once the incision has been made, an anterior skin flap is raised between the parotid gland capsule and superficial fat layer. The platysma, medially, and greater auricular nerve, laterally, can be used to identify the correct plane inferiorly. The flap over the parotid gland can be raised using a blade or scissors. Good retraction helps identify the plane to prevent a breach through the skin, gland or tumour capsule. As the anterior border of the parotid gland is reached care must be taken to prevent damage to branches of the facial nerve as they emerge from the gland. The flap is retracted anteriorly with sutures.

The sternocleidomastoid muscle is identified and its anterior border dissected free. The greater auricular nerve will be encountered. It is sometimes possible to preserve a posterior branch that supplies sensation to the ear lobe. The posterior belly of the digastric muscle is exposed and traced back to its insertion in the mastoid. The perichondrium of the tragus is identified and the tragus exposed to its deep extent to reveal the tragal pointer. Another suture retracts the ear lobule posteriorly. The parotid gland between the tragus and posterior belly of digastrics is carefully dissected to ensure wide exposure.

There are several ways to find the facial nerve. A combination of the first three landmarks is usually adequate to ensure safe dissection in the majority of cases:

1 Finding the nerve as it bisects the tympanomastoid groove. This is the most constant landmark.
2 Using the tragal pointer, the nerve lies approximately 1 cm deep and 1 cm inferior to the nerve. The nerve lies just deep and superior to the posterior belly of digastric near its attachment to the mastoid.
3 Where a large tumour lies directly over the proximal aspect of the facial nerve, find a distal branch, such as the marginal mandibular, and follow the nerve in a retrograde manner.
4 Where the above measures fail, drill into the mastoid portion of the temporal bone to

identify the descending portion of the facial nerve and follow it out of the stylomastoid foramen.

Careful dissection on a broad front with precise use of bipolar diathermy to ensure complete haemostasis will allow identification of the facial nerve trunk (Figure 26.3), which can be confirmed by use of a nerve stimulator. The main trunk typically divides into upper and lower divisions, which divide in a variety of combinations into the five terminal branches. There is often some cross-communication between the branches. Each branch of the facial nerve is followed using a small, curved clip to dissect the gland from the nerve, ensuring that no pressure or compression of the nerve occurs, which would result in postoperative weakness. The gland may then be cut superficial

to the nerve under direct vision using a No. 12 scalpel, scissors or electrosurgery device (e.g. ligasure). Bipolar diathermy must be used precisely to prevent thermal damage to branches of the facial nerve.

Parotid tumours often lie directly over branches of the nerve. Care is taken not to enter the tumour, as this risks recurrence at a later date.

The parotid gland is carefully dissected free of the facial nerve, preserving all branches. Very rarely, when no other option is available, typically due to malignancy, one or more branches of the facial nerve may have to be sacrificed. A drain is usually required and an absorbable suture used to close the platysma, with the skin closed with a non-absorbable monofilament suture or staples.

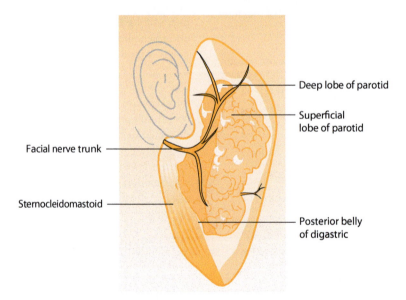

Deep lobe of parotid

Superficial lobe of parotid

Facial nerve trunk

Sternocleidomastoid

Posterior belly of digastric

Figure 26.3. Identification of the facial nerve trunk.

POSTOPERATIVE REVIEW

Always check and document facial nerve function postoperatively and exclude a haematoma. The drain will usually be left in place at least overnight. The patient can be discharged home once the drain has been removed.

Sutures or skin staples are removed at 5–7 days, with a follow-up arranged to review histology in the clinic.

27 TRACHEOSTOMY

Francis Vaz

A tracheostomy is a conduit from the skin of the neck to the trachea. It is classically performed in an open surgical fashion, however, more recently percutaneous techniques have been developed and are frequently used. The formation of an open surgical tracheostomy may be required in the emergency or elective setting.

Indications

- Real or anticipated airway obstruction.
- Prolonged ventilation.
- Pulmonary toilet.

METHODS

Thyroid cartilage

Cricothyroid membrane

Cricoid cartilage

First tracheal ring

Site of tracheotomy

- *Cricothyroidotomy* – This may be required in the emergency setting when access to the airway is required. The gap between the thyroid and cricoid cartilages (cricothyroid membrane) is palpated. A horizontal stab incision facilitates the insertion of a mini-tracheostomy.
- *Percutaneus tracheostomy* – This technique has gained popularity with intensive therapy unit (ITU) interventionists. It is performed using a Seldinger technique where a guide wire is inserted through a transtracheal needle which has been placed in the midline through the skin into the trachea. A series of dilators are gradually 'railroaded' over this to widen the tract. Finally, the tracheostomy tube can be inserted.

This is often performed with the benefit of a flexible bronchoscope through the larynx from above to ensure correct positioning in the trachea.

- *Transtracheal needle* – Wide-bore needles are available which can be inserted and then connected to a jet ventilation system to maintain an airway. This is a temporary measure to allow oxygenation while a secure airway is inserted.
  Since it does not allow for expiration, the upper airway should be clear enough to allow for gases to be expired.
- *Surgical tracheostomy* – This will be considered in greater detail below.

FORMATION OF A SURGICAL TRACHEOSTOMY

A tracheostomy is usually performed under general anaesthesia, although the use of local anaesthesia may be necessary where the airway is too narrow to allow intubation. The skin is infiltrated with local anaesthetic and the tracheal mucosa injected just before an incision is made into the trachea.

The procedure requires the following steps:

1 *Patient position* – The patient is positioned supine with the head in the midline. A sandbag is placed under the shoulders and a head ring is used to support the head. This extends the neck allowing the laryngeal skeleton and trachea to be readily palpated and elevated into the neck.
2 *Skin incision* – A skin incision is made halfway between the cricoid and the suprasternal notch and extended into the subplatysmal tissues (Figure 27.1). The anterior jugular veins and midline strap muscles will now come into view (Figure 27.2).
3 *Identification of the thyroid gland and trachea* – The strap muscles are separated in the midline and retracted, bringing the trachea and thyroid isthmus into view (Figure 27.3).
4 *Division of the thyroid gland* – The thyroid gland is clamped through the isthmus, divided

in the midline and a transfixion suture used to prevent bleeding. With the thyroid isthmus divided, the trachea will be better exposed. A single tube may be chosen at this point, but a variety of sizes should be available. The tube cuff should be checked for leaks at this point.

5 *A window into the trachea is fashioned* – Inform the anaesthetist before entering the trachea. There are a number of methods of entering the trachea. In children, a vertical slit is made in the midline and stay sutures placed on either side of the incision. These sutures are taped to the child's chest and used to hold open the hole if the tracheostomy tube displaces or when the tracheostomy tube is first changed at seven days. In adults, a window is cut just large enough to admit the tracheostomy tube. In both cases the cricoid cartilage must not be injured. For this reason, the window or incision is made through the 2nd, 3rd or 4th tracheal rings (Figure 27.4).
6 *A tracheostomy tube is inserted* – Ask the anaesthetist to deflate the cuff and withdraw the endotracheal tube until the tip is just above the window. The tracheostomy tube may be inserted, the cuff inflated and the tube sutured into place and appropriate dressings applied.

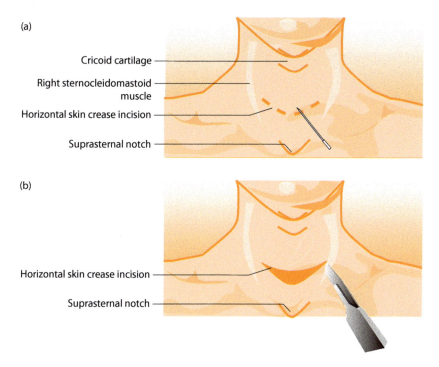

(a)

Cricoid cartilage

Right sternocleidomastoid muscle

Horizontal skin crease incision

Suprasternal notch

(b)

Horizontal skin crease incision

Suprasternal notch

Figure 27.1. Tracheostomy incision.

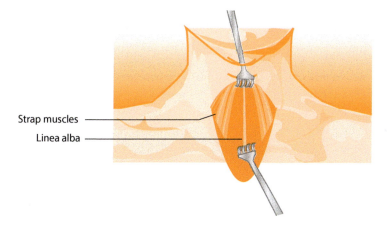

Strap muscles

Linea alba

Figure 27.2. Identification of thyroid isthmus.

If an emergency tracheostomy is required, it is essential to gain access and maintain the airway as quickly as possible. In these cases, a vertical midline incision is made to avoid all vascular structures except the thyroid, which must be dealt with rapidly in the emergency scenario.

Complications

These may be classified as immediate, early and late.

Immediate (within 24 hours of procedure)
Haemorrhage — thyroid vessels, jugular veins.
Pneumothorax.
Air embolism.

First tracheal ring

Thyroid isthmus

Fourth tracheal ring

Figure 27.3. Division of thyroid isthmus.

First tracheal ring

Window

Figure 27.4. Tracheal window.

Cardiac arrest
Local damage to thyroid cartilage, cricoid
  cartilage, recurrent laryngeal nerve(s).
Dislodgement or displacement of the tube.

Early (24 hours–7 days)
Dislodgement or displacement of tube.
Surgical emphysema of neck.
Crusting.

Infection.
Tracheal necrosis.
Tracheoarterial fistula.
Tracheooesophageal fistula.
Dysphagia.

Late (after 7 days)
Tracheal stenosis.
Difficulty with decannulation.
Tracheocutaneous fistula.

TRACHEOSTOMY TUBE CARE AND SPEAKING VALVES

Tracheostomy tube care is often left to tracheostomy nurse specialists or members of the nursing staff. It is, however, essential that junior doctors are able to care for patients with tracheostomy tubes in place and are aware of the potential complications of having a tracheostomy. It is often the case that out-of-hours emergencies and advice will be directed towards the junior on-call surgeon.

At their bedside, all patients should have a spare tracheostomy tube of the same size and one smaller, a tracheal dilator, a 10 mL syringe, a suction unit and catheters, gloves, Spencer Wells forceps and lubrication for the tubes.

▌ Tracheostomy tubes

- Cuffed.
- Uncuffed.
- Fenestrated.
- With or without an inner cannula.
- Adjustable flange.
- Suction assisted.

A tracheostomy tube can be directly attached to an anaesthetic circuit provided that there is a 15 mm connector at the proximal end. Some tubes have this segment on the inner tube, so this should always be available.

Cuffed tubes (Figure 27.5)

Advantages:

- A cuff is required for:
  - Ventilation, continuous positive airway pressure.
  - Patients who aspirate as they cannot protect their airway.

Patients with normal swallowing reflexes may find their swallowing impaired as a result of pressure exerted on their oesophagus and the impedance of laryngeal elevation by an inflated cuff.

Disadvantages:

- If the tube lumen becomes blocked, the patient's airway is compromised leading to respiratory arrest as there is no capacity to breathe around the tube, unless the cuff is deflated.
- The cuff can damage the tracheal mucosa, leading to ulceration and possible stenosis. Rarely, however, this may also cause arterial erosion.
- Children younger than 10 years, have a narrow trachea, and unlike in an adult, the larynx is conical, with the cricoid cartilage forming the narrowest segment. Tracheostomy tubes used in children are uncuffed.

$$\text{Pressure} = \text{Force/Area}$$

Low-pressure, high-volume cuffs reduce the incidence of pressure-induced complications, but it is still important not to over-inflate the cuff.

The cuff should be deflated as soon as possible to allow for the insertion of a speaking tube or decannulation cap.

Uncuffed tubes (note Figure 27.6)

These tubes are often found in patients returning from ITU after a prolonged stay as they allow

Flange

Outer tube

Inflated cuff

Obturator tip

Figure 27.5. A cuffed tracheostomy tube.

suction and physiotherapy. The tubes are easy to replace and suitable for long-term use. Patients can speak around it. They are not suitable for patients who aspirate or who need ventilation.

Fenestrated tubes

The fenestration directs airflow through the patient's vocal cords, oropharynx and nasopharynx. It helps some patients to resume breathing normally and can be used to wean them off their tracheostomy tube. Remember that a fenestrated inner tube is also required.

Tube with adjustable flange

This is designed for patients with deep-set tracheas and fat necks.

The flange can be adjusted to fit the depth of tissue between incision and trachea.

▌ Cleaning inner tubes

Most recommend water or warm salty water only. Avoid alcohol, bleach and glutaraldehyde. Flush the tube and do not soak it as this increases the risk of bacterial proliferation.

Humidification

- Nebulizers 5 mL, 0.9% N/saline in mask over stoma.
- Heat moisture exchangers fit onto the tracheostomy tube.

- Foam filter protectors such as the Buchanan laryngectomy protector.

▌ Tracheostomy dressings

The objective is to keep the trachea, stoma and adjacent skin clean and dry, and minimize skin irritation and infection. Wet skin results in maceration and excoriation. Hydrophilic polyurethane foam dressings absorb moisture away from the skin.

If a tracheostomy site shows signs of granulation, this can be treated with silver nitrate cautery, although care should be taken not to damage surrounding normal skin.

▌ Changing a tracheostomy tube

Most surgeons recommend the first tube change to be performed at 1 week. The first change should be performed by an experienced practitioner or, ideally, by the surgeon.

If a difficult tube change is anticipated, use an exchange device (guide wire or a bougie) and consider changing the tube in the operating theatre.

The steps involved are as follows:

1 Explain to the patient what you plan to do. Ensure that a good light source, preferably a headlight, is available.

Tape
Flange

Figure 27.6. Tracheostomy tube in situ.

2 Extend the patient's neck using pillows so the head is supported and hyperoxygenate them if required.
3 Check the integrity of the cuff if used. Lubricate it sparingly.
4 Remove all old dressings and clean around the stoma site.
5 Remove intraoral secretions with suction, deflate the cuff and suction through the old tube. Some secretions trapped around the cuff will now fall into the trachea inducing coughing.
6 Allow the patient to recover and remove the old tube.
7 Insert a new tube, inflate the cuff if indicated and insert the inner cannula.
8 Check chest movement, insert a clean dressing and apply the tapes before checking cuff pressure.
9 If you are uncertain of the position of the tube, a flexible endoscope can be passed into the trachea through the tube lumen.
10 Connect to any humidification devices.

GENERATING A VOICE WITH A TRACHEOSTOMY

- Cuff deflation.
- Fenestrated tracheostomy tube (and inner tube).
- Smaller tracheostomy tube.
- Intermittent finger occlusion.
- One-way speaking valves.

All of the above allow air to escape around or through the tube into the larynx and the oropharynx. One-way speaking valves allow air to be inspired but not exhaled through the tube.

Do not put a one-way speaking valve on patients with a cuffed fenestrated tube unless their inner tube is also fenestrated. If you do, they will struggle.

It can take time for patients to get used to a speaking valve, and they need to be encouraged to breathe in through their tracheostomy and out through their mouth. Patients need to be monitored for signs of respiratory distress in the early stages of using a one-way speaking valve.

Contraindictions

- End-stage pulmonary disease.
- Excessive secretions.
- Unstable medical.
- Anarthria.
- Unstable ventilatory status.
- Airway obstruction.
- Severe anxiety or cognitive dysfunction.
- Severe tracheal or laryngeal stenosis.
- Inability to tolerate cuff deflation.

28 VOICE

Francis Vaz

Voice is the method by which humans predominantly communicate. However, speech also allows us to add emotion and expression to what we communicate. Changes in our voice, therefore can alter the way we communicate or express ourselves.

The production of voice, however, is not purely based around the larynx, as it is essential to have the 'ballast' from the lungs to produce the vibration created at the laryngeal level. This vibratory source creates a sound that is shaped and moulded by the articulators and resonators in the upper aerodigestive tract (UADT). A change in any of these three areas can change the quality of the voice.

The vibratory source creates a sound by chopping up air from the trachea by the intricate movement of the vocal cord mucosa. The vocal fold is a five-layered structure that allows the mucosa to move over Reinke's space and the lower elements that make up the vocal fold ligament. This movement is referred to as the mucosal wave, and it forms a vibration that is then moulded by the UADT. The vocal folds may vibrate 80–1000 times/second; therefore, if visualized with white light, the mucosal wave cannot be visualized. Stroboscopic examination allows for the production of a montage of different phases in the cycle of the mucosal wave to be collected and visualized on screen. This chapter deals specifically with the history, examination and subsequent management of patients with abnormalities of the larynx.

HISTORY

When taking a history it is essential to listen carefully to the voice itself, as often a diagnosis can be made by listening to the quality of the voice and the story that comes with it.

It is essential to find out what the patient uses their voice for — both in their occupation and in their hobbies.

Certain professions put more strain on voices (e.g. teachers and actors) and are prone to pathology as a result.

The duration and progression of the hoarseness are important to ask about as longstanding voice changes are unlikely to be sinister, but a progressive change in the voice over a few months, especially associated with other UADT symptoms such as dysphagia, odynophagia, a neck mass or otalgia, indicates a potential malignant pathology.

Preceding symptoms, such as an upper respiratory tract infection (URTI) can affect the likelihood of pathology forming, especially in a situation where the voice is strained as a result of the URTI.

A thorough medical and drug history should be taken to assess conditions that may affect the ballast (respiratory drive) to produce voice. Also, certain medications may affect voice as they may precipitate coughing (angiotensin converting enzyme inhibitors [ACEIs]) or may dry the UADT (e.g. anticholinergic side effects).

EXAMINATION

Initially, a general ENT examination is helpful, specifically to look at the oral cavity, oropharynx and nasal cavity, because these are the articulators and resonators and therefore affect voice.

Laryngeal examination then follows. The voice clinic often uses rigid laryngoscopy or flexible nasolaryngoscopy with a stack system.

A stroboscopic light source allows the mucosal wave to be captured and processed by the human retina, enabling visualization of the differences between mucosal waves and also pathologies. Without a strobe the vibrations of the mucosal wave are too fast for the human retina to register. The strobe splits the wave up and puts together a cycle of its different aspects in a slower fashion for the retina to distinguish.

PATHOLOGY

Voice changes at the laryngeal level occur because of the following changes:

1 Mass effect on the vocal fold.
2 Incomplete closure of the vocal folds.

3 Poor vibration or mucosal wave as a result of pathology.

Common voice conditions and their treatment options are described below.

REINKE'S OEDEMA

In this situation the patient has had a long-standing deepening of the voice. They are often smokers, but acid reflux may also play a part. Pathologically, oedema occurs within Reinke's space in the vocal fold, increasing the mass of the vocal fold and therefore deepening the voice (Figure 28.1).

The correct treatment is smoking cessation and the use of anti-reflux therapy in the form of a proton pump inhibitor. If the patient ceases smoking but the voice does not return to normal and the findings are still the same on laryngoscopy, then a superior cordotomy on the non-vibratory surface of the vocal cord can be undertaken and some of the oedema reduced.

VOCAL FOLD NODULES ('SINGER'S' NODULES)

These are often associated with actors or singers, although professional singers often have an excellent understanding of their voice and do not often present with nodules. Often the strain of pushing one's voice in inappropriate scenarios (i.e. acting or singing) can strain the voice and lead to trauma

and the formation of nodules. Others (e.g. teachers and instructors in a noisy environment such as a swimming pool) may also suffer.

The larynx often shows bilateral nodules at the junction of the anterior third and posterior

Figure 28.1. Cross section of the vocal cords.

two-thirds. This does not allow for good closure of the vocal folds and results in a change in voice.

For the vast majority of these we use speech and language therapy to educate patients on use of the voice and to help them use their voice appropriately. Rarely do they require surgical intervention.

VOCAL FOLD PALSY

Patients present with a recent onset, 'breathy' voice which becomes tired with use. The two vocal folds do not meet because one vocal fold is immobile and therefore a lot of air escapes and a breathy voice is created.

Sinister aetiology should be excluded as the nerve supply to the larynx is from the vagus via the recurrent laryngeal nerve. Imaging, including the skull base through to the upper chest, should be undertaken for a left cord palsy as the recurrent laryngeal nerve descends to the aortic arch on this side, and from skull base into the root of the neck for a right cord palsy (CT scan ± MRI skull base).

Initially for an idiopathic vocal fold palsy speech and language therapy should be undertaken to see if the patient can compensate for the immobility and make the other cord come across further to make more contact and improve the voice. If this fails, or for malignant aetiology (e.g. terminal lung cancer damaging the recurrent laryngeal nerve), speedier intervention is necessary. This requires an injection thyroplasty to medialize the immobile vocal cord, either as an outpatient or under general anaesthetic. An alternative is to medialize the vocal cord externally using a piece of silastic or Goretex through a window in the thyroid cartilage.

LARYNGEAL CANCER

These patients usually present with a long history of smoking and/or high alcohol intake. They

have developed a progressively worsening voice over 6–12 weeks and may have associated otalgia, odynophagia, dysphagia and even associated neck lymphadenopathy.

Nasoendoscopy usually demonstrates an irregularity of the vocal fold, but the patient requires a laryngoscopy and biopsy of this suspicious area.

In smokers a premalignant diagnosis of dysplasia may be made on histology. This is just as important, as the patient needs to be aware of this and to stop smoking to reduce the chance of progressing to an invasive malignancy. Prior to biopsy a staging computed tomography of the neck and chest is useful.

Laryngeal cancer can be treated in a variety of ways. Small laryngeal cancers can be treated with narrow field radiotherapy or be resected using a laser at the time of laryngoscopy. Larger tumours can be treated with radiotherapy or chemo-radiotherapy covering a larger field for associated lymph nodes. The largest laryngeal cancers – those that have invaded the thyroid cartilage and those that may be obstructive to the airway — are often treated with a laryngectomy. This involves removal of the larynx and the creation of a permanent end stoma. The management of the patient should be discussed in the context of a multidisciplinary head and neck team meeting.

LARYNGEAL PAPILLOMATOSIS

Human papilloma virus (HPV) can cause viral warts. In the larynx this can be extremely troublesome. If a viral wart impinges the glottis, the airway may be compromised, but more often hoarseness is produced due to incomplete closure of the glottis and/or poor mucosal wave formation.

There are many treatments. Surgical interventions are often reserved for significant airway

obstruction or for significant change in voice due to mass effect. The problem is that each surgical procedure is associated with some laryngeal scarring, and although some patients will require multiple procedures it is wise to minimize the trauma to the larynx unless there is good reason to operate on it.

HAEMORRHAGIC POLYP

This pathology is not infrequently seen following an upper respiratory tract infection, where the voice has been used and then a small telangiectatic vessel bleeds. This slight irregularity on the vocal

cord leads to a change in voice. This sometimes heals, but occasionally persists and matures. If persistent, it may require surgical excision with a microlaryngoscopy with or without laser resection.

VOCAL CORD GRANULOMA

Patients typically have undergone recent surgery requiring endotracheal intubation or have been on the Intensive Care Unit with an endotracheal tube in situ for a few days. The pathology forms typically on the posterior medial aspect of the

vocal cord over the vocal process of the arytenoid cartilage.

The granuloma forms due to healing exposed cartilage as a result of trauma from an endotracheal tube. Also of importance in the pathology may be gastropharyngeal reflux of acid.

Treatment often involves aggressive anti-reflux treatment over a 6-week period, but if symptoms and signs persist, surgical resection may be undertaken with a micro-laryngoscopic technique.

VOCAL CORD CYSTS

This pathology presents clinically with a change in voice, but it can be very variable in its severity and frequency. It may relate to the actual type of vocal cord cyst, as some are superficial mucosal cysts and some are deeper intracordal cysts. These can be very difficult to treat and should be managed in a dedicated voice clinic, with full speech and language therapy support. However, if surgery is to be considered, it should be carefully undertaken, raising a microflap, dissecting the cyst out and causing minimal mucosal trauma. This should not be underestimated, as it can prove to be a significant surgical challenge.

MICROLARYNGOSCOPY

This is an examination under general anaesthesia and is often undertaken for diagnostic or therapeutic procedures on the larynx. The use of the microscope offers magnification, depth of field, bimanual handling of instrumentation and the use of other attachments, such as a CO_2 laser.

Before commencing a laryngoscopy the patient should be placed in 'the sniffing the morning air' position, which is flexion of the neck and extension of the atlanto-occipital joint. A decision on how to maintain the airway should be made with the anaesthetist (i.e. with a micro-laryngoscopy tube, supraglottic/subglottic or transtracheal jet ventilation).

The endoscope, light source, suction, lubrication and dental guard should all be checked prior to starting with the laryngoscopy. The laryngoscope is inserted carefully to get a view of the larynx and then suspended with a Lewis suspension arm. At this point the microscope or a Hopkins rod may be used for more careful examination of the larynx in preparation for the biopsy or surgical undertaking.

29 AIRWAY MANAGEMENT

Francis Vaz

Airway management is one of the most critical emergency situations in ENT practice. A sound understanding of the anatomy, physiology and management of a patient with airway problems is essential. In light of the order of resuscitation priorities — Airway, Breathing, Circulation (ABC) – the importance of airway management cannot be underestimated.

An additional point to consider is that as the airflow increases through a narrowed segment, pressure is decreased. This is known as the Bernoulli's phenomenon. This draws the mucosa into an already narrowed airway inducing local oedema of the mucosa, which further narrows the airway with resulting compromise.

A further point to note is the difference between an adult's airway and a child's. In the child, the airway is both absolutely and relatively smaller than in the adult. The larynx is higher and external landmarks are less easily identifiable. The trachea lies nearer the skin in children, diving into the chest at a steeper angle than in the adult. Important contents of the thorax (e.g. the domes of the lungs and the great vessels) lie higher in the child. In addition, since the neonate is an obligatory nasal breather, nasal obstruction resulting from bilateral choanal atresia may be fatal.

MANAGEMENT OF THE COMPROMISED AIRWAY

Presentation and management of the compromised airway varies according to the site of presentation and aetiology (Table 29.1). These affect both the severity and speed of onset of symptoms and the categorization of management into urgent or nonurgent. However, the approach taken to manage airway obstruction is similar for all.

It is essential in the management of the patient with a compromised airway that a team approach is used. The most senior members of the anaesthetic and ENT teams should be informed and involved in the management at an early stage.

More than one option or plan should be discussed before significant intervention is undertaken.

A rapid assessment of the patient is made to assess whether they are in danger of imminent upper airway obstruction. This is determined by the worsening of stridor or stertor, although stridor that becomes quiet may indicate imminent complete airway obstruction.

Stertor is rough noisy breathing, similar to snoring, caused by vibration of partially obstructing soft tissue in the pharynx.

Table 29.1. Aetiology of airway obstruction.

Level of obstruction	Aetiology	
	Pathological	**Anatomical**
Nasopharynx	Tumour Infection Foreign body	Choanal atresia (unilateral or bilateral) Crouzon syndrome Apert syndrome
Oropharynx/ Hypopharynx	Infection (tonsillitis, Ludwig's angina) Bleeding (post-tonsillectomy) Tumour Burns Trauma Anaphylaxis	Short lower jaw (especially micrognathia) Large tongue
Supraglottis	Infection (epiglotitis, supraglottitis) Bleeding Tumour (squamous cell carcinoma, respiratory papillomatosis) Cyst of vallecular or epiglottis Anaphylaxis Foreign body	Laryngomalacia
Glottis	Infection (croup) Tumour (squamous cell carcinoma, respiratory papillomatosis) Vocal cord palsy Polyp Oedema (postoperative anaphylaxis) Foreign body	Laryngeal cleft Laryngeal web
Subglottis	Infection (croup) Tumour (squamous cell carcinoma, respiratory papillomatosis) Stricture (post-intubation, post-tracheostomy) Extrinsic compression (thyroid, lymph nodes, tumour) Foreign body	Congenital subglottic stenosis Subglottic haemangioma
Tracheal	Infection (tracheitis) Tumour (squamous cell carcinoma, respiratory papillomatosis) Stricture (post-tracheostomy) Foreign body Bleeding (post-tracheostomy) Burns	Tracheosophageal fistula

Stridor is a harsh, high-pitched, almost musical sound, caused by vibration of partially obstructing soft tissue in the larynx or upper trachea.

Inspiratory stridor is during inspiration only, often a crowing sound, and is due to obstruction at the glottis, supraglottis or subglottis level.

Expiratory stridor is during expiration only, usually at a slightly lower pitch than inspiratory stridor, and is due to obstruction of the subglottis or extrathoracic trachea.

Biphasic stridor involves both inspiration and expiration, and, while representing laryngeal obstruction, is a hallmark of severe obstruction.

Wheeze is a high-pitched husky or whistling sound, caused by narrowing of soft tissue in the intrathoracic airways.

In addition, patients will have a high respiratory rate, poor chest expansion, low oxygen saturations, tachycardia and may experience fatigue with rising carbon dioxide. While it may be possible in an adult to examine the larynx using a flexible nasoendoscope in order to assess the degree of obstruction, this must not be attempted in a child. When presented with a child with imminent airway compromise, such as suspected epiglottitis, any instrumentation may cause significant distress and a decline in the airway. The priority is to secure the airway, ideally in theatre. It is very rare that a patient presents in complete airway obstruction. In this case, it is likely that an anaesthetist will already be with the patient. If they are unable to intubate the patient, then an immediate tracheostomy must be performed in order to secure the airway. This is described in Chapter 27.

Immediate management includes calling for senior help, and giving oxygen and adrenaline nebulizers. Heliox can also buy valuable time. It is composed of 21% oxygen and 79% helium and has a lower density than air, which improves flow in the airways resulting in better oxygen delivery. The administration of steroids gives benefit a few hours later by reducing mucosal oedema. If in the emergency room, the patient should be monitored in the resuscitation area. If patients are stable, they are managed in a high dependency or critical care unit. Where a patient is not severely compromised, a more thorough evaluation may be made, including appropriate imaging and a plan made depending on the aetiology.

If the patient is in complete airway obstruction or, despite the above measures, continues to deteriorate, then a decision must be taken to secure the airway with a cuffed endotracheal tube. Ideally, this should be performed in the operating theatre where all the anaesthetic equipment for managing difficult airways is available, as well as the surgical instruments for tracheostomy and rigid bronchoscopes.

A plan is made jointly by the senior ENT surgeon and anaesthetist to determine how they will secure the airway. This depends on the suspected level of obstruction. Orotracheal or nasotracheal intubation may be attempted by the anaesthetist if it is thought that there is sufficient space to pass a tube through the obstruction safely. The surgeon and scrub nurse must be scrubbed with tracheostomy and bronchoscopes open and set up in order to intervene if needed. Other temporary airway adjuncts that should be considered to gain access to the subglottis include a transtracheal cannula or cricothyroidotomy with jet ventilation. If intubation fails or is thought not to be possible, then the decision is taken either to perform a tracheostomy or gain initial access to the airway by bronchoscopy with a rigid ventilating bronchoscope.

Table 29.1 is a summary of the most common aetiologies that can result in airway obstruction, along with the level of obstruction.

KEY POINTS:

- A is for airway, and the presentation of an acutely problematic airway is a medical and surgical emergency.
- Act sooner rather than later, especially if you suspect a progressive problem.
- Consider medical management that may be of use to hold the situation without causing the patient distress (adrenaline nebulizers, steroids, heliox).
- Involve senior members of the ENT, anaesthetic and if appropriate nursing/paediatric teams as soon as possible.
- Think before you act, as you may precipitate a worsening of the problem.

30 RADIOLOGY

Dipalee Durve and Kaggere Paramesh

LATERAL SOFT TISSUE FILM

This is a plain x-ray performed in the acute setting for investigation of an ingested foreign body in an adult or child. A normal lateral soft tissue film is illustrated in Figure 30.1.

Always check for prevertebral soft tissue swelling.

The maximum normal width anterior to the upper cervical vertebral bodies (C1—C4) should measure up to 7 mm. The maximal normal width increases to 22 mm in the lower cervical vertebrae (C5—C7).

This is more easily estimated by remembering that up to a third of the vertebral body is allowed between C1—C4 and a whole vertebral body's width is allowed anterior to C5—C7.

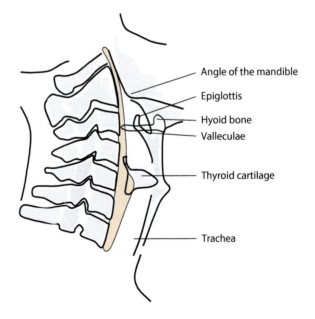

Angle of the mandible
Epiglottis
Hyoid bone
Valleculae
Thyroid cartilage
Trachea

Figure 30.1. Landmarks visible on a lateral soft tissue film of the neck. The soft tissue space anterior to the vertebral column should always be inspected.

There is a wide variety in the radio density of swallowed foreign bodies. Whilst some ingested foreign bodies are radio-opaque and clearly visible on a lateral soft tissue film, many are not. Helpful secondary radiological signs that suggest the presence of an impacted foreign body include widening of the prevertebral soft tissue space (as a result of surgical emphysema due to perforation or retropharyngeal abscess formation), tenting of the cervical oesophagus producing a gas shadow in the upper cervical oesophagus or straightening of the normal cervical lordosis.

Common sites for impingement of chicken or fish bones include the palatine tonsils, tongue base, valleculae and pyriform fossae. The oesophagus is narrowed just below the level of the cricopharyngeus and at the level of the aortic arch. It is here that foreign bodies are commonly located.

A normal soft tissue lateral film cannot exclude a radiolucent foreign body and a low threshold should be maintained for endoscopy. Similarly, normal variants with calcification within the cricoid or arytenoids can be mistaken for bones due to their curvilinear calcification.

A chest x-ray may be an alternative test if the suspected level of the obstruction is in the thoracic oesophagus or airways.

Common sites of oesophageal foreign body impaction are:

- At the level of the cricopharyngeus.
- Where the arch of the aorta indents the oesophagus.
- Where the right main bronchus indents the oesophagus.
- At the cardiac sphincter.

CONTRAST SWALLOW

A contrast swallow may be indicated for the following:

- Globus sensation.
- Suspected pharyngeal pouch.
- Suspected foreign body.
- Suspected oesophageal lesion.

The barium or contrast swallow is a fluoroscopic technique using low-dose pulsed x-rays to examine the pharynx and oesophagus. It can be used to demonstrate strictures, tumours, pharyngeal pouches, tracheo-oesophageal fistulae, oesophageal dysmotility and gastro-oesophageal reflux. A non-ionic contrast medium such as Omnipaque is used in cases where there is a clinical suspicion of aspiration as barium can remain in the chest indefinitely and alternatives such as gastrograffin can cause a chemical pneumonitis.

ULTRASOUND NECK

Ultrasound is a safe, easily accessible test. Superficial structures such as the thyroid, parotid and submandibular glands are easily evaluated and beautifully depicted. Morphology of lymph nodes and the presence of any suspicious features (Table 30.1), as well as diagnostic fine needle aspiration (FNA), can be performed (1). The presence of collections and whether they would be amenable to drainage can be determined. In children it can be used to assess lesions such as thyroglossal cysts or fibromatosis colli (sternomastoid tumour). The presence or absence and velocity of coloured blood flow in congenital lesions such as venolymphatic malformations and haemangiomas can be assessed as an adjunct to further cross-sectional imaging, such as MRI.

Table 30.1. Morphology of lymph nodes in the neck.

	Benign lymph node	Malignant lymph node
Size	Variable; reactive lymph nodes can be very large in the neck.	Size alone cannot be used to differentiate benign vs malignant. Increase in nodal size in a patient with known malignancy is suspicious for involvement.
Shape	Elliptical (short to long axis ratio of <0.5).	Round (short to long axis ratio >0.5).
Border	Usually not sharp borders.	Sharp borders – due to intranodal tumour infiltration causing increase in acoustic impedance between node and surrounding tissues. However, metastatic lesions in advanced stages may have ill-defined borders due to extracapsular spread of tumour.
Echogenicity	Intermediate echogenicity.	Usually hypoechoic relative to adjacent musculature. However metastatic nodes from papillary thyroid carcinoma usually hyperechoic due to intranodal deposition of thyroglobulin.
Echogenic hilum	Usually seen in nodes >5 mm.	May be absent due to tumour infiltration but can also be seen in malignant nodes. Therefore cannot be used as sole criterion for evaluation of neck nodes.
Intranodal necrosis	Not seen.	May be cystic (liquefaction necrosis) or echogenic (coagulation necrosis). Found in metastatic and tuberculous lymph nodes and regardless of nodal size should be considered pathological.
Calcification	Usually not seen.	Some cancers, e.g. papillary or medullary thyroid cancers, can have calcification, usually peripheral, punctate with acoustic shadowing.
Vascular distribution	Hilar vascularity.	Peripheral or mixed vascularity.

COMPUTED TOMOGRAPHY AXIAL VIEWS OF THE NECK

Computed tomography (CT) of the neck is usually performed in the acute setting for assessing adenopathy or a collection. MRI is better at delineating soft tissue planes and has no ionizing burden, but availability in the acute setting is limited, and scanning times can be lengthy for the improved spatial resolution required for the small structures in the neck.

COMPUTED TOMOGRAPHY OF THE TEMPORAL BONE

CT of the temporal bone is used as a preoperative planning tool in cases of cholesteatoma where disease spread resulting in bony erosion is particularly significant (Figure 30.2). The bony ossicular chain and inner ear can be assessed as well as the aeration of the surrounding mastoid air cells. It is also useful in cases where hyperostosis is seen as a complication of meningitis.

Figure 30.2. (a−g) Axial CT views of the right temporal bone (superior to inferior).

A CT scan is reviewed in order specifically to assess:

- Extent of disease.
- Pneumatization of the temporal bone.
- Position of the sigmoid sinus.

- Facial nerve dehiscence.
- Position and dehiscence of the tegmen/middle fossa plate.
- Ossicular chain continuity.
- A breach of the inner ear.

CT OF THE SINUSES

CT of the sinuses has now replaced plain film radiography and is indicated in patients who do not respond to medical treatment of sinusitis. It can demonstrate severity and distribution of disease, patency of the osteomeatal complexes and any anatomical variants such as concha bullosa (an accessory air cell within the middle turbinate), Haller and Onodi cells and to aid surgery. Both axial sections and coronal reformats are required.

A CT scan is reviewed in order specifically to assess:

1 Extent of disease.
2 Position of the septum — a deviated septum may require correction in order to access the paranasal sinuses (Figure 30.3).
3 Position of lamina papyracea and uncinate process.
4 Attachment of the middle turbinate.
5 Presence of a concha bullosa.
6 Length of the lateral lemniscus (Keros classification; Table 30.2).
7 Position of the optic nerves (axial views).

Anterior ethmoidal air cell
Lamina papyracea
Uncinate process
Maxillary sinus
Septum

Lateral lemniscus
Middle turbinate
Inferior turbinate

Figure 30.3. Coronal section of the paranasal sinuses.

Table 30.2. The Keros classification refers to the vertical height of the lateral lemniscus. Types 2 and 3 are at greater risk of cerebrospinal fluid leak during functional endoscopic sinus surgery.

	Vertical height of the lateral lemniscus
Type 1	1–3 mm
Type 2	4–7 mm
Type 3	8–16 mm

MAGNETIC RESONANCE IMAGING

Indications

- Assessment of the tongue base.
- Assessment of parotid lesions.
- Intracranial pathology (e.g. cerebellopontine angle lesions).

MRI is increasingly used in the head and neck due to its capacity to image soft tissues. This modality remains the investigation of choice in the assessment of tongue base or parotid lesions. In the case of the latter, the retromandibular vein allows one to distinguish between the larger superficial and smaller deep lobe tumours. The extent of tongue carcinoma is best defined radiologically with particular regard to whether the midline has been crossed, whether there is involvement of the mandible, and any spread posteriorly to the epiglottis.

Most ENT surgeons will request this investigation for cases of asymmetric sensorineural hearing loss (>15 dB HL difference in two adjacent frequencies), sudden sensorineural hearing loss and unexplained vertigo or dizziness. It may also be used to assess patients with delayed or absent recovery of a facial nerve paralysis.

This investigation is contraindicated in patients with metal foreign bodies and implants (e.g. pacemakers, cochlear implants, etc.).

Both high-resolution CT and MRI are important in the investigation of congenital deafness as well as the surgical planning of any treatment. There is a wide range of anatomical abnormalities, some linked to syndromes, including the Mondini spectrum and widening of the vestibular aqueduct.

▌ MRI IAMs

Normal anatomy, including the VIIth and VIIIth nerve roots and the vestibular aqueduct, are exquisitely demonstrated (note Figure 30.4).

Figure 30.4. Normal MRI view of the internal auditory meatii (see Chapter 1, Figure 1.5 regarding the relative positions of the nerves within the internal auditory meatus).

POSITRON EMISSION TOMOGRAPHY – COMPUTED TOMOGRAPHY IMAGING (PET-CT)

PET has the ability to detect abnormal metabolic activity at cellular level in organs that do not yet appear morphologically different on other imaging modalities.

▍ Uses of PET-CT in head and neck malignancy

PET-CT is useful in giving physiological and anatomical information and particularly important in detection and follow-up of head and neck tumours.

PET-CT is used for:

● Detection of recurrent disease:
  – Neck dissection and flap reconstruction distort normal anatomy making detection of recurrent disease very difficult on CT alone.

– Radiation therapy causes oedema making tissue planes indistinct, also difficult to detect recurrence.
● Detection of recurrence of cranial base neoplasms.
● Directing biopsy.
● Detection of unknown primary tumour site:
  – Cervical node metastases common with occult carcinoma.
  – PET-CT used to detect areas that are PET-avid and may be a source of the malignancy (Figure 30.5).
● Staging head and neck tumours.

PET-CT pitfalls (2):

● Physiological FDG uptake – normal in several head and neck areas and may cause false positives.
● Recent surgery.

Figure 30.5. (a) CT and (b) PET-CT fused with PET avid nodes in supraglottic SCC.

- Recent radiation and chemotherapy.
- Inflammatory tissue.
- Tumours with low FDG avidity e.g. salivary gland and necrotic neoplasms can cause false negative results.

REFERENCES

1 Ahuja, W. et al. 2008. Ultrasound of malignant cervical lymph nodes. *Cancer Imag* 8: 48–56.
2 Meltzer et al. 2005. Combined PET-CT in head and neck – diagnostic uses and pitfalls. *Radiographics* 25(4): 913–30.

31 MANAGEMENT OF NECK LUMPS

Francis Vaz

The management of masses in the head and neck region may seem daunting because of the wide variety of pathology and the consequences of missing an important diagnosis. This exceptionally common clinical finding can be seen across age groups and important factors must be elicited in order to obtain the correct diagnosis.

An understanding of the anatomy of the neck and the associated pathologies relevant to the various positions in the neck is helpful. Delineation of whether a lump is in the midline (often suggestive of a thyroid or thyroglossal cyst pathology) or laterally, either in the anterior or posterior triangle of the neck, can assist in the diagnosis (Table 31.1).

Table 31.1. General considerations in the diagnosis of a neck lump.

Age (yrs)		Position
<20	Inflammatory	Midline – Thyroglossal cyst
	Congenital	Dermoid
	Lymphoma	Lymph node
20–40	Salivary disease	Thyroid
	Thyroid disease	Lateral – Lymph node
	Inflammatory	Salivary
	Malignancy	(upper)
>40	Malignancy	

HISTORY

A careful history should be elicited from the patient. Age of onset of the neck lump should be documented as congenital pathology presents in the early years and more often malignant pathologies present later in life. Upper aero-digestive tract symptoms, such as dysphonia, dysphagia, odynophagia, otalgia and breathing disorders, can be helpful in localizing pathology. Personal habits such as smoking and high alcohol intake can highlight a risk for malignant potential.

EXAMINATION

A thorough examination of the head and neck should be undertaken. The oral cavity should be illuminated with a headlight and examined with two tongue depressors. If appropriate, the tongue base should be palpated as pathology may be deep and not obvious to the eye (this does, however, induce a significant gag reflex). A flexible fibreoptic nasolaryngoscope is usually required to assess the postnasal space, larynx and hypopharynx. Any masses in the neck should be identified in a careful and methodical examination of the neck.

SPECIAL INVESTIGATIONS

The use of special investigations can be divided into those pertinent to preparing a patient for a general anaesthetic and those relevant to the pathology of the head and neck.

When investigating a lump in the neck the principal investigation of choice, almost always, is fine needle aspirate cytology (FNAC). This is a process by which cells are sampled by means of multiple passes of a needle through the mass while simultaneously aspirating with a syringe. The cells in the barrel of the needle are then sprayed onto a cytology slide and either air-dried or fixed chemically, depending on the preference of the cytology department. This test is often undertaken by the cytology department itself. This is a crucial investigation and there are only a few instances where an FNAC of a neck lump is not appropriate.

Imaging of masses in the neck is commonplace. The choice of imaging is dependent on the patient and the institution where it is to be performed.

Ultrasonography is an excellent, noninvasive tool to delineate structures but is difficult for the surgeon to interpret. Computerized tomography (CT) is superb for looking at most of the head and neck, is easy to obtain and quick to undertake, but can be prone to dental artifacts in and around the oral cavity. Magnetic resonance imaging (MRI) is an excellent tool to look at soft tissues, especially of the tongue, postnasal space and oral cavity. It does often carry a longer waiting time to be performed, is more claustrophobic to undertake, and takes longer to be scanned.

Investigations pertinent to general anaesthesia should be discussed at a local pre-admission level, and each department should have an appropriate protocol for preparing a patient for general anaesthesia.

TREATMENT

The treatment of any neck mass is dependent on the diagnosis. Reactive lymphadenopathy secondary to tonsillitis requires treatment of the tonsillitis with antibiotics. Congenital pathologies may be observed if asymptomatic but, if causing problems, often warrant surgical excision. The primary malignant disease of the upper aero-digestive tract may be treated with surgery, radiotherapy, chemoradiotherapy or a combination of these. All treatment plans will be decided in the context of a multidisciplinary team meeting.

LYMPHADENOPATHY

Lymphadenopathy can be benign or malignant. The benign causes of lymphadenopathy are multiple and too large a group to be discussed in this chapter. However, a lymph node in the neck should be approached as though it is malignant until it is shown that it is not.

Our index of suspicion is changed by different aspects of the history, clinical examination, and special investigations performed. Metastatic lymphadenopathy typically follows a predictable path dependent on the primary site of the tumour (Figure 31.1). This should be borne in mind when searching for the primary tumour. Lymphoma is a diagnosis that should be considered, but is difficult to diagnose on FNAC. Often a lymph node biopsy/core biopsy is required for formal exclusion or typing of the lymphoma.

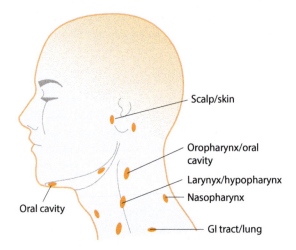

Figure 31.1. Metastatic spread from primary sites in head and neck cancer.

THYROGLOSSAL DUCT CYST

This congenital anomaly occurs due to residual portions of the tract that forms during the descent of the thyroid gland during embryological development. The cysts can form at any point along the descent of the thyroid and are often found in a paramedian position, between the trachea and the base of tongue.

These should be investigated with an ultrasound scan to look at the mass, but also to check for a normal thyroid gland, as surgical excision is often contemplated and one must be certain that there is other thyroid tissue left behind after its removal.

Surgery is in the form of a Sistrunk procedure or midline neck dissection, clearing the tissue from the midline of the neck and the cyst whilst taking out the mid-portion of the hyoid bone. Removal of the mid-portion of the hyoid bone is undertaken due to the intimacy of the embryological descent with the hyoid, and its removal significantly decreases the recurrence rate of these cysts.

BRANCHIAL CYST

Branchial cysts are another congenital pathology that typically present in the first two decades of life. They may present as an asymptomatic mass, but can be seen to enlarge, especially in association with upper respiratory tract infections. The position of these is quite characteristic, being hidden under the junction of the upper third and lower two-thirds of the sternocleidomastoid muscle.

FNAC often demonstrates a straw-coloured liquid. Imaging should be undertaken in the form of a CT or MRI scan of the neck to give relationships to the great vessels and also to characterize the mass further.

Surgical excision should not be undertaken lightly and should be considered almost like a selective neck dissection, such that the accessory, hypoglossal and vagus nerves are identified and preserved, together with the internal jugular vein and the carotid artery.

THYROID MASSES

Thyroid masses are commonplace and warrant a whole chapter. However, certain aspects of the history should be elicited, namely aspects of the lump and growth rate, pain, dysphagia, hoarseness and stridor, together with aspects of risk factors, such a family history or exposure to ionizing radiation.

Many people argue about investigation of the thyroid mass. This depends on the institution's expertise; however, most people with a mass in the thyroid will have at least an ultrasound ± FNAC to guide surgeons in their management plan.

Treatment is dependent on the appearances of the FNAC and ultrasound, together with the patient's feeling about the lump, as cosmesis is potentially an indication for removal of the goitre.

SALIVARY GLAND TUMOURS

This is an extensive subject, but it is useful to have an understanding of it.

Eighty percent of salivary gland tumours arise in the parotid, 10% in the submandibular gland and 10% in the sublingual or minor salivary glands. Of the parotid tumours, 80% are benign and, of these, 80% are pleomorphic adenomas.

Hallmark symptoms and signs of malignant pathology include rapid growth of mass, pain and nerve weakness (e.g. facial nerve weakness in parotid malignancies).

FNAC is very useful and can be very helpful in the decision-making process for these tumours.

32 VERTIGO AND DIZZINESS

Rahul Kanegaonkar

Vertigo and dizziness affect approximately one third of the general population before the age of 65 years (1). Annually, five out of every thousand patients present to their general practitioner complaining of symptoms classified as vertigo, with another ten per thousand with symptoms of dizziness or giddiness (2). A balance disorder in the elderly may result in a fall, with the subsequent injuries sustained leading to serious injury and even death.

BALANCE OVERVIEW

Normal human balance function relies on vision, the peripheral vestibular organs, proprioception and hearing (Figure 32.1). This sensory information is relayed centrally, where it is integrated and interpreted within the brain in order to maintain posture, stabilize vision and provide information regarding self and environmental movement (spatial awareness). Interpretation involves cross-referencing this sensory information with previously generated templates. A mismatch results in symptoms of dizziness, unsteadiness or vertigo.

HISTORY

Taking a thorough history is the key to establishing a diagnosis. It is essential to allow patients to speak freely at the start of the consultation. Although some of this information may be of little diagnostic value, it does allow some insight into their principal concerns and also establishes rapport with the individual patient. It is often the case that this will be the first time that 'anyone has listened'.

A detailed history of the first episode is essential. When, where and what possible precipitants were associated with the event should be sought (e.g. had the patient rolled over in bed, a recent change in medication). The duration and form of dizziness/vertigo should also be established. Associated symptoms should be documented (e.g. nausea, vomiting, hearing loss, tinnitus, loss of consciousness, photophobia and headache).

Subsequent episodes, their duration, frequency and precipitants will confirm a working diagnosis. The most recent episode is also worth exploring as symptoms may evolve as central changes partially compensate for the peripheral or central pathology. It is always worth considering more than a single pathology responsible for a patient's symptoms (e.g. benign paroxysmal positional vertigo (BPPV) and a peripheral vestibular deficit).

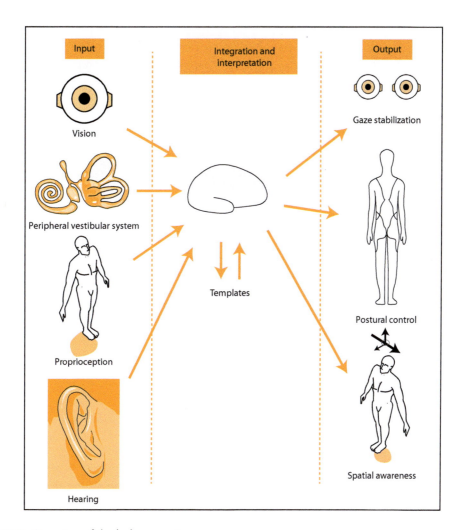

Figure 32.1. Overview of the balance system.

A past medical and surgical history must always be taken, including details regarding the patient's vision and mobility and a family or personal history of migraine. In females, a delicate and difficult subject is that of spontaneous miscarriage, but may suggest an autoimmune or embolic aetiology.

EXAMINATION

A neuro-otological examination is required in every patient presenting with vertigo. Although a working diagnosis may have been made, it is essential both to confirm and exclude possible concurrent pathology. This includes ear and cranial nerve examination, eye movement in all four planes for nystagmus, smooth pursuit, saccades and latent squint and cerebellar signs. Romberg test (on both floor and foam) and the Fukuda stepping test should also be performed. Whilst the latter is generally regarded to localize a peripheral vestibular deficit (rotation occurs towards the weaker side), the Halmagyi head thrust test is a far more sensitive and specific clinical investigation (Table 32.2). Dix–Hallpike testing is also required in every case to demonstrate any form of nystagmus, but in particular geotropic torsional nystagmus consistent with posterior semicircular canal BPPV. Vertical or horizontal nystagmus, or nystagmus that does not fatigue, is unusual, and patients require MRI scanning to exclude central pathology. It is essential to document the latency and duration of any nystagmus seen and whether the nystagmus settled completely.

A thorough assessment also includes lying and standing blood pressure recording and gait assessment.

SPECIAL INVESTIGATIONS

All patients should undergo a pure tone audiogram and tympanometry. A sensorineural asymmetry may suggest a cerebellopontine angle tumour, which must therefore be excluded with MRI internal auditory meatii. Vestibular testing is required in the majority of subjects referred to a balance service (exceptions may include BPPV that settles completely following particle repositioning manoeuvres). Not only do these investigations support a working diagnosis, but in approximately 5%–10% of cases reveal unexpected unilateral or bilateral peripheral vestibular hypofunction and guide vestibular rehabilitation.

As it is not possible to directly access the peripheral vestibular organs, an indirect assessment based on the vestibulo ocular reflex is generally used (Figure 32.2).

Bithermal caloric testing remains a simple and valuable method of comparing lateral semicircular canal function. Eye movements may be recorded with electrodes attached to the face, electronystagmography (ENG) or by videoing pupil movement, videonystagmography (VNG). Saccades, smooth pursuit and optokinetic movement may also be assessed with this recording method. Additional tests include rotational chair and vestibular evoked myogenic potentials (VEMPs).

Patients with a history and assessment in keeping with central pathology should also undergo an MRI scan to exclude a space-occupying lesion or demyelination. Patients with chronic ear disease or suspected superior semicircular canal dehiscence require a fine-cut computed tomography scan of the temporal bones.

COMMON VESTIBULAR PATHOLOGY

Listed below are common vestibular conditions amenable to treatment (Table 32.1). Management pathways are also illustrated in Figure 32.3.

▌ Benign paroxysmal positional vertigo (BPPV)

This is the commonest cause of vertigo in all age groups. Patients classically describe rotatory vertigo when rising or turning over in bed. Although the vertigo lasts for seconds, they feel unsteady for a great deal longer, but are then able to go about their normal daily activities. There is no associated hearing loss or tinnitus. Spells last for days to weeks and usually settle spontaneously. Patients often describe a previous head injury, episode of 'labyrinthitis' or a brief spell of environmental tilting ('the floor suddenly came up to meet me').

Symptoms arise due to debris derived from the otoconial membrane of the utricle. Head rotation results in this debris striking the delicate cupula of the posterior semicircular canal, profoundly

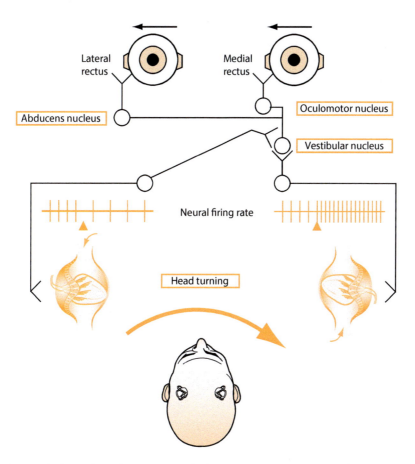

Figure 32.2. The vestibulo ocular reflex. As a result of head rotation, endolymph flow within the semicircular canals causes movement of the cupulae within the ampullae of the lateral semicircular canals and relative shearing of the underlying stereocilia. Neural impulses increase on the right and decrease on the left. Neural connections to the IIIrd and VIth cranial nuclei result in contraction of the left lateral rectus and right medial rectus to stabilize gaze.

Table 32.1. Common causes of dizziness (in order of frequency).

- Benign paroxysmal positional vertigo (BPPV)
- Acute peripheral vestibular deficit (labyrinthitis/vestibular neuritis)
- Vertiginous migraine
- Multilevel vestibulopathy
- Cholesteatoma (CSOM)
- Hyperventilation syndrome
- Menière's disease
- Vestibular schwannoma
- Multiple sclerosis
- Vertebrobasillar insufficiency
- Superior semicircular canal dehiscence

stimulating the associated hair cells and causing vertigo (Figure 32.2). The mismatch in input between each side that occurs may also result in nausea, vomiting and anxiety.

The most common form affects the posterior semicircular canal. On Dix–Hallpike testing, following a short latency, geotropic (towards the ground) torsional nystagmus will gradually appear, increase in severity and gradually subside completely. This will correlate well with the symptoms of vertigo experienced by the patient during the test. Having confirmed the diagnosis, an Epley manoeuvre should be performed. This

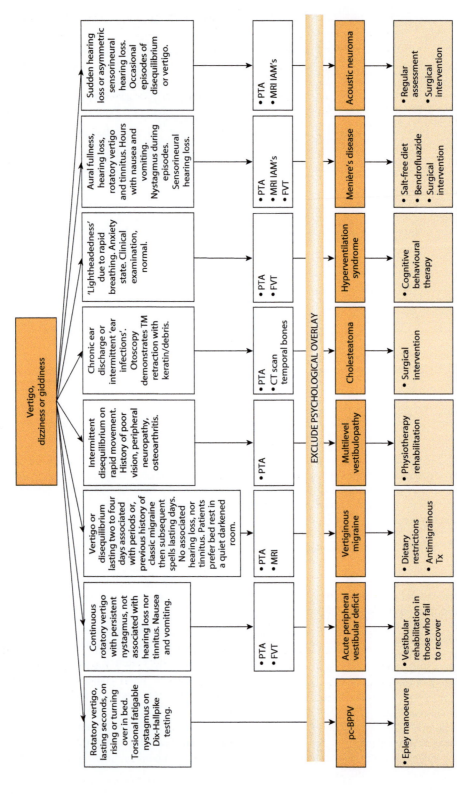

Figure 32.3. Management pathways for common vestibular pathology. (PTA – pure tone audiometry; FVT – formal vestibular testing)

is curative in approximately 90% of cases. A repeat manoeuvre may on occasion be required. Alternative particle repositioning manoeuvres for posterior semicircular canal BBPV include Brandt–Daroff (9) and Semont manoeuvres (10). Gans manoeuvre may be used if the anterior semicircular canal is involved (11).

▌ Acute peripheral vestibular deficit (labyrinthitis/vestibular neuritis)

This relatively common cause of vertigo arises due to a sudden failure of one peripheral vestibular organ. This results in labyrinthine asymmetry, and the sensory mismatch that occurs causes severe persistent rotatory vertigo and profuse vomiting.

Patients may describe a recent flu-like illness. They classically wake up with severe continuous rotatory vertigo that persists for 3–5 days. Initially, patients must lie still as any movement results in worsening symptoms. Thereafter, movements may be tolerated, but compensation for normal activities may take weeks or months. Prochlorperazine, a peripheral vestibular sedative, is indicated in this situation, but should be limited to 7 days, as long-term use may limit central compensation and, hence, functional recovery.

Clinical examination may reveal rotation on Fukuda. More reliable is the head thrust test, where a catch-up saccade may be evident (note Table 32.3).

Table 32.2. Limitations of vestibular compensation.

Visual impairment	Cataracts Poor visual acuity Eye movement disorders
Peripheral vestibular system	Prolonged vestibular sedative use (e.g. prochlorperazine)
	Recurrent or progressive vestibular insults
Proprioception	Immobility
Psychological factors	Anxiety Depression Agoraphobia
Central pathology	Cerebrovascular disease Intracranial pathology
Rehabilitation	Delay in starting vestibular rehabilitation Poor motivation

Patients who do not compensate benefit from generic or customized physiotherapy. Those with visual vertigo (over-reliance on visual input) benefit from combining physiotherapy exercises and visually stimulating environments (12). Those who fail to improve must be reassessed and possible limitations to compensation excluded (Table 32.2).

Table 32.3. The sensitivity and specificity of clinical tests used to identify peripheral vestibular hypofunction.

Clinical test	Sensitivity (%)	Specificity (%)
Gait assessment	23–86	38–92
Halmagyi head thrust test	34–100	64–100
Head shake test	35–95	62–92
Romberg test	61–79	58–80
Stepping tests	50	61
Dix–Hallpike testing for PC-BPPV	79	75

▌ Vestibular migraine

Also known as vertiginous migraine, this common cause of vertigo produces spells of vertigo or disequilibrium that last for several days and, in women, are frequently cyclical as they are hormone related. Patients often describe phonophobia or photophobia and prefer to rest in a quiet, darkened room. This is not usually associated with hearing loss or tinnitus.

Although no abnormalities are likely to be found on clinical examination, ENG/VNG testing may support central changes. All patients should undergo MRI scanning in order to exclude central pathology.

Treatment consists of dietary changes (avoidance of chocolate, caffeine, red wine, cheese and processed meat). The majority of patients benefit from this approach alone, although some may also require tricyclic antidepressants, calcium channel blockers or beta-blockers.

▌ Multilevel vestibulopathy

Dizziness and vertigo are common symptoms in elderly patients.

Unilateral decline in one sensory pathway may be compensated for centrally, with little or no functional loss. A reduction in the quality and quantity of sensory information from multiple sensory pathways (e.g. worsening vision, proprioceptive loss due to diabetes mellitus), in addition to central changes within the brain (e.g. ischaemic episodes) may result in multilevel vestibulopathy. Patients benefit from a combination of physiotherapy exercises (generic, customized or strength and balance exercises) and lifestyle changes (e.g. the use of a walking stick, glasses or cataract correction).

▌ Cholesteatoma (CSOM)

Squamous epithelium within the middle ear may expand to erode into the inner ear. While most patients present with intermittent or chronic ear discharge and hearing loss, some also experience intermittent vertigo and unsteadiness.

▌ Hyperventilation syndrome

Hyperventilation associated with anxiety, may result in lightheadedness and dizziness. In some, anxiety may be the residual effect of a previous vestibular insult that the patient may have compensated for. Asking a patient to breathe rapidly through pursed lips can reproduce symptoms. These patients benefit from cognitive behavioural therapy.

▌ Ménière's disease

Often misdiagnosed, this very uncommon cause of vertigo arises due to expansion of the scala media compartment within the inner ear. As a result Reissner's membrane may intermittently rupture resulting in mixing of perilymph and endolymph and toxic over excitation of the neuronal elements within the inner ear.

Attacks are unpredictable and severe. An initial feeling of aural fullness is followed by hearing loss, severe rotatory vertigo and tinnitus. A pure tone audiogram will demonstrate a sensorineural hearing loss, initially in the low frequencies in the affected ear and then, as attacks continue, hearing loss across all frequencies. It is essential to exclude a central pathology (e.g. a cerebellopontine angle tumour) and, hence, an MRI scan must be performed. Bithermal calorics will reveal a peripheral vestibular weakness. Attacks eventually subside but at the expense of the hearing in the affected ear.

Treatment includes sublingual prochlorperazine for acute episodes, and bendrofluazide or betahistine to reduce the frequency and severity of attacks.

For those not controlled medically, surgery may be indicated. Procedures include grommet insertion, transtympanic gentamicin ablation, labyrinthectomy and vestibular nerve section. Up to 50% of patients may develop bilateral disease. Bilateral vestibular hypofunction results in severe oscillopsia, with patients wheelchair-bound and unable to move their heads. Hence, vestibular destructive procedures should be avoided if possible.

OTHER CAUSES

Other relatively uncommon conditions that may present with vertigo or dizziness include multiple sclerosis, vestibular schwannoma (Figure 32.4), and vertebrobasilar ischaemia. In each an MRI scan is required to establish a diagnosis.

Superior semicircular canal dehiscence is a rare condition whereby a defect in the bony covering of the superior semicircular canal results in a third window through which a pressure wave may be transmitted from and into the intracranial cavity. This not only results in momentary vertigo in response to loud sounds (Tullio's phenomenon) but also results in patients hearing their eyes moving.

Figure 32.4. Right vestibular schwannoma.

KEY POINTS:

- An understanding of the sensory pathways and their central interpretation provides a valuable guide to the diagnosis and management of patients who complain of vertigo and dizziness.

- While a number of conditions exist that may result in vertiginous spells, treatment is either curative or enormously beneficial in the vast majority of patients.

- The commonest cause of vertigo, BPPV, should be excluded in all cases by Dix–Hallpike testing.

REFERENCES

1 Shepard NT, Telian SA (1996a). *Balance Disorder Patient. Basic Anatomy and Physiology Review*. Singular Publishing Group, Inc.

2 The Royal College of General Practitioners and Office of Population Census and Surveys (1986). Morbidity Statistics from General Practice. HMSO, London.

3 Blake AJ, Morgan K, Bendall MJ et al.(1988). Falls by elderly people at home: Prevalence and associated factors. *Age and Ageing* 17: 365–72.

4 Campbell AJ, Reinken J, Allan BC, Martinez GS (1981). Falls in old age: A study of frequency and related clinical factors. *Age and Ageing* 10: 264–70.

5 Stevens JA, Olson S (2000). Reducing falls and resulting hip fractures among older women. *MMWR Recomm Rep* 49: 3–12.

6 McKenna L, Hallam RS, Hinchcliffe R (1991). The prevalence of psychological disturbance in neurootology outpatients. *Clinical Otolaryngology* 16: 452–6.

7 Halmagyi GM, Curthoys IS (1988). A clinical sign of canal paresis. *Archives of Neurology* 45: 737–9.

8 Dix, R, Hallpike C (1952). The pathology, symptomatology and diagnosis of certain common disorders of the vestibular system. *Annals of Otology, Rhinology and Laryngology* 6: 987–1016.

9 Brandt T, Daroff R (1980). Physical therapy for benign paroxysmal positional vertigo. *Archives of Otolaryngology* 106: 484–5.

10 Semont A, Freyss G, Vitte E (1988). Curing the BPPV with a liberatory maneuver. *Advances in Otorhinolaryngology* 42: 290–3.

11 Gans R (2000). Overview of BPPV: Treatment methodologies. *Hearing Review* 7: 50–4.

12 Pavlou M, Lingeswaran A, Davies RA et al. (2004). Simulator based rehabilitation in refractory dizziness. *J Neurol* 251: 983–95.

INDEX